LEARNING STRATEGIES

A PRACTICAL GUIDE TO THE
DEVELOPMENT OF STRATEGIC LEARNERS

Learning Strategies The Missing 'Think' In Physical Education And Coaching

A Practical Guide To The Development Of Strategic Learners

Andy Anderson, PhD
Ontario Institute for Studies in Education
University of Toronto

Sport Books Publisher

Canadian Cataloguing in Publication Data

Anderson, Andy Thomas
    Learning strategies: the missing 'think' in physical education and coaching: a practical guide to the development of strategic learners

Includes bibliographical references.
ISBN 0-920905-66-8

1. Physical education and training—Study and teaching. 2. Learning strategies. I. Title.

GV363.A52 2001   613.7'071   C00-932252-3

Summary: The book is designed to prepare learners in physical education, recreation, and athletic settings to think more precisely and critically about their own thinking, feelings, and actions. Learning strategies enable learners to think things through: "What am I supposed to do? How can I prepare myself to do this well?" Strategy use should empower students to engage actively in the learning process, to understand more about learning in general and to appreciate their own capacities as a learner. Most importantly, strategy use should help build stronger self-confidence among students.

Distribution worldwide by Sport Books Publisher

http://www.sportbookspub.com
E-mail: sbp@sportbookspub.com
Fax: 416 966-9022

Printed in the United States

Acknowledgements

I would like to express my sincere thanks to a number of people who helped put this text together:

To my publisher and his staff, who provided invaluable assistance in helping to shape the book.

To my daughter, Alanna, who has always helped me 'think' more deeply about everything.

To my wife, Bonnie, for her continued support of all my endeavours.

Contents

Chapter 4　**Imagery 55**

Chapter 5　**Self-talk 77**

Contents cont.

Preface

Physical education should equip students with the essential knowledge and skills that will enable them to lead healthy lives now and in the future. If students are expected to function on their own, schooling must prepare them to acquire, analyze, and apply new information in diverse situations. Instruction must not only help students achieve their immediate learning goals, but also prepare them to manage learning situations effectively beyond school.

This book aims to assist those who teach physical education or coach young athletes in better preparing students to become deliberate, responsible, flexible, and productive learners. By focusing on instructional practices grounded in cognitive research, students are able to construct a deeper understanding of the learning process, advance their understanding of movement, and develop the habits of mind associated with life-long learning (e.g., attentiveness, searching for meaningful patterns, strategic and fluent thinking, finding and keeping focus).

Cognitive instruction emphasizes learner involvement in the learning process. This work synthesizes and distills findings from researchers at both the university and school levels to pinpoint the most effective teaching methods for implementing strategy instruction in physical education. In so doing, this book provides practical guidance to school professionals who desire to design instruction promoting strategic learning, but who do not have the opportunity to participate in intensive training programs offered as a part of specific strategy instruction programs.

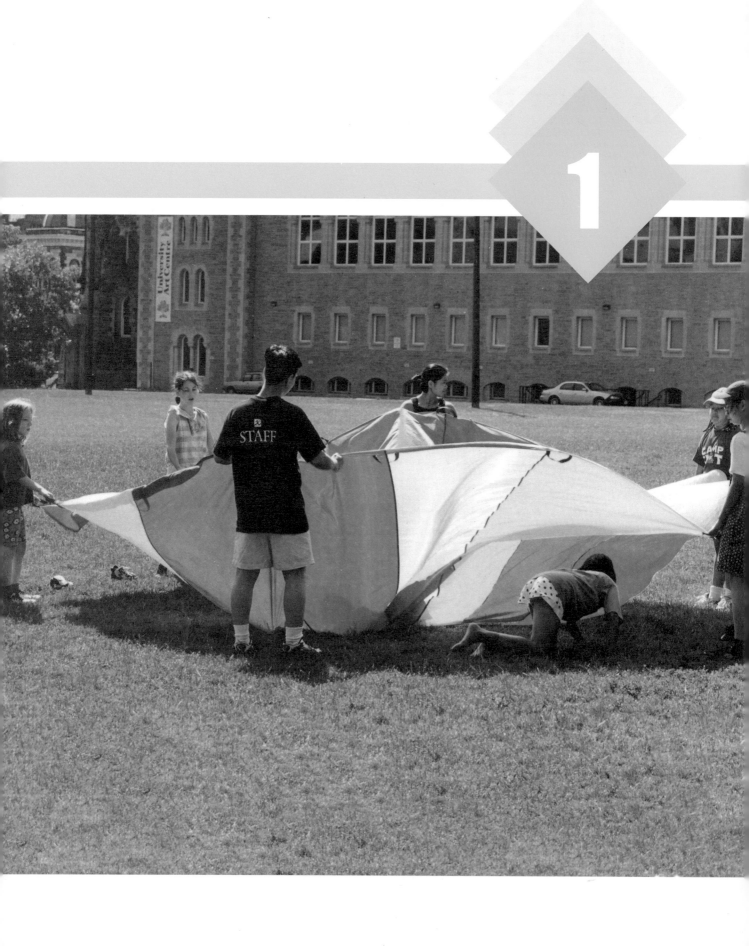

1

INTRODUCTION TO THE BOOK

Chapter Outline

- ◆ **Who Will Benefit From This Book?**

- ◆ **Beliefs and Assumptions That Guide the Structure of the Book**

- ◆ **Why the Missing 'Think'?**

- ◆ **Learning by Observation**

- ◆ **Benefits of Strategy Use**

- ◆ **How to Use This Book**

Chapter Objectives

Recognize the significance of learning strategy use in physical education settings

Identify beliefs that underlie the book

Identify benefits of strategy use in physical education

Education is an active attempt by the learner to make sense of instruction and experience. Learning is an interpretive, creative process.

You need tools if you plan to build something.

This book is about learning strategies – what they are, why they are important, and how students can use them to become more proficient and self-reliant learners. Learning strategies are the mental tools used systematically to manage the thought processes associated with knowledge and skill acquisition (Anderson, 1997).

Skilled performers (mountain climbers, carpenters, painters, surgeons) use a variety of cognitive tools (the analysis of and application of knowledge and skills to new situations) and meta-cognitive tools (the planning and monitoring of progress and outcomes) to increase both efficiency and effectiveness. The tools used to promote learning are powerful only when they are used properly. Tools do not create the finished product. The degree to which a person uses the 'right' tools the 'right' way determines whether the outcomes achieved are worthwhile and satisfying. Tool management is both science and art. Creativity and technique go hand-in-hand in preparing and executing skilled actions. The ability to use a variety of learning tools in a variety of ways advantages both the performer and performance.

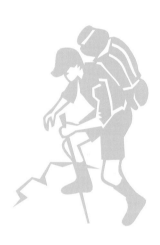

Tool selection and application are an integral part of any goal-oriented process. Mountain climbers do not randomly select their equipment; equipment use is planned carefully considering the direction of the climb, anticipated challenges, and the skill of the climber. Similarly, learners must have a clear sense of where they are going, the route they intend to follow, obstacles they encounter (fear, embarrassment, self-doubt), and the strategies that will enable them to deliberately achieve their goals while avoiding and coping with difficulties and setbacks.

The benefits of a strategic approach to task attainment are obvious. Strategic learners are deliberate and resourceful about their thinking, intended actions, performances, and emotions before, during, and following instruction and practice. Strategic learners make it happen. It is important, however, to understand how each strategy works for the learner personally, how to use the strategy flexibly and creatively, and under what conditions each strategy is most likely to benefit individual performance.

This book is organized to give teachers and students the background knowledge and learning experiences related to four learning strategies: picture words, imagery, self-talk, and goal-setting. This work originated from research conducted in classrooms (Anderson, 1992) and from scholarship that focused on training elite athletes. However, the ideas presented here have been designed specifically for use in the regular physical education programs.

High performance athletes have enjoyed the benefits of mental training. Dwight Stones drew the world's attention to mental rehearsal in the 1976 Olympics in Montreal. Before each jump, we could see him preparing for the jump with his head bobbing through the approach and the lift over bar. He performed this ritual not once but several times before he actually executed the jump. His results were golden. There is no evidence to suggest beginners could also not benefit from use of mental training techniques to overcome the complexities of learning a new skill. If it is indeed possible to improve both rate and retention in learning, then mental training should become a routine part of the physical education program. In fact, as I will point out later, in order to effectively achieve the primary goals of physical education (e.g., commitment and capacity to lead a healthy active life), learning strategies must be a central and fundamental part of the learning process (i.e., developing the capacity to learn on your own).

The essential message of this book is that strategic learners:

♦ can and are willing to do more on their own to improve

♦ feel better about the results because they 'own' the skill

♦ engage persistently and confidently in new learning challenges

Who Will Benefit From This Book?

This book is for teachers and coaches interested in having learners assume greater control over and responsibility for their own learning. Students should benefit most from this book since they will become better able to purposefully and deliberately perform the learning tasks.

Beliefs and Assumptions That Guide the Structure of the Book

1. Strategy use should be an integral part of self-control (the ability to regulate thought and action) and self-reliance (the sense that the individual can exercise control over their thoughts and actions).

2. All children can learn most of the skills taught in physical education if they are taught in a way that enables them to assume control over the learning process.

3. Skill development is enhanced when students know more about the mental activities associated with skill acquisition (e.g., vividly picturing the activity before trying it is a good way to focus and rehearse the movement).

4. The ability to relate thought and action to solve problems is a mark of intelligence.

Why the Missing 'Think'?

The problem is not that students do not think; it is that children may not think about the 'right' thing or with the 'right' tools to make appropriate decisions about how to perform well. The 'think' that is missing is the thinking that is associated with deliberate practice. Focused, planned, purposeful, and consciously aimed at improving the key features of performance, deliberate practice involves the intentional choice of a particular strategy to execute tasks at a higher cognitive level. The drive towards excellence requires long hours of practice. Unless learners are 'on track' cognitively, emotionally, and physically, they may be simply going through the motions, failing to make important and continuous gains. Those who are focused on the task learn faster, develop higher levels of proficiency, retain that proficiency longer, and can transfer it to new learning challenges (Landin, 1994; McCullagh & Scheid, 1995; Stiehl & Weiss, 1990). Strategic learners are also better prepared to engage in independent tasks and are more likely to be better prepared for a lifetime of physical activity.

Learners may think skill achievement is the result of luck - "either it happens or it doesn't" or genetic endowment - "he's good at that because he is a boy" or "his dad was good that's why he's so good, too." Unless learners are taught to focus on the subtleties of a particular action, given the tools to manage that information appropriately and strategically, and encouraged to think in resourceful ways about how to improve their skills, long hours of practice may result in little (if any) improvement, bad habits, frustration, and unfulfilled potential. On the other hand, learners taught to engage strategically in the development of skills become more resilient, efficacious, and persistent— and, as a result, more highly skilled.

Learning by Observation

In most instances, learners rely on observation to gather information about how to perform specific tasks. Although important, watching a performance is often not enough. For example, while a magician performs on the stage, the audience participates in the illusion by focusing on the show - the presentation and the outcome. What the observers are directed to pay attention to are details that seldom have anything to do with the trick. Unless the audience is privy to the performer's thinking we remain baffled, but entertained.

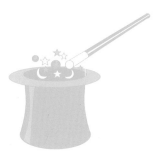

Similarly, students tend to focus on performance outcomes – how far, how hard or how high the ball travels – versus the key features of a quality performance that generate the intended outcomes – *"begin by standing sideways, extend the arms like wings of an eagle, rock back,"* etc. Learning strategies should be seen as tools used to enhance mental acuity and to foster the emotional stability required for optimal physical performance during the early stages of learning and throughout the learner's life.

Benefits of Strategy Use

1. Too often, the teacher or other students do the thinking for the learner, creating a cycle of dependence. The longer students depend on others, the more likely they will continue to remain dependent thinkers and problem-solvers, both in school and beyond. In other words, if students are not prepared to lead their own lives (intellectually, socially, morally, physically, emotionally, and spiritually), they will be lead by others.

2. If educators can enhance the learner's chances of success, they should. The more children experience success in school programs, the more likely they are to improve their skills during their spare time, and perhaps prolong their involvement in physical activity beyond their school years.

3. Much of a student's motor development is acquired through practice that occurs outside school time. The opportunities students have to receive immediate, constructive, reflective feedback are limited. There are often too many students in class, too little time for instructors to interact with students one-on-one, and too few scheduled classes to administer frequent and individual feedback. Preparing students to monitor their own progress and to work with their peers are powerful ways of providing feedback in the absence of teachers or coaches.

4. Rather than relying on the teachers as the final arbitrators of quality, evaluation responsibilities can be assumed by the students themselves. Learners are shown the highest level of respect when they are enabled to become "artisans of their own learnings and doings" (Hawkins, 1974, p. 48) - in other words, when they are prepared to become their own teachers.

5. Self-study and self-challenge are major parts of maturation and competency development. Self-study is more than independent study of a given subject. It is reflective and critical understanding of learning. Self-study entails several key questions. For example: what do I know already? how do I know what I know? how can I move to the next level of performance? what tools do I have to improve? what kind of information and how should that information be represented for me to understand it? who or what are trustworthy sources of information? how will I know when I have moved to the next level?

How to Use This Book

Competent and confident use of learning strategies occurs best when instruction and practice are combined to make informed decisions. Teachers and coaches should customize strategy use to suit each individual and his/her particular circumstances. The best way to teach learning strategies is to describe their nature, proper use and benefits, and to model their use so that students will have concrete images of the strategy in action. Allow students time in and outside class to explore strategy use as it occurs in everyday situations; urge them to discuss strategy use with their parents and friends.

It is important also for students to understand that strategy use should be an integral part of learning. Always connect strategy use to understanding more about the skill development and about the learning process itself. Students also need to appreciate that strategy use enhances control over thinking, emotions, feelings and to understand how these are connected to skill development.

Spend time each class talking about the strategy, its occurrence in class, and in other situations outside class. Encourage students to share their ideas, insights, and stories about strategy use. Display the situations and the uses of strategy described by students in chart form. Show that their ideas count and can contribute to the knowledge about learning and strategy use. Students can also keep journals or portfolios with descriptions of how they improved a given skill.

Both teachers and students must be curious and inventive about strategy use. Although there are descriptions for how to use each strategy in the chapters that follow, don't be afraid to adapt them to your specific situation or for particular student needs and interests. Take note of how students choose to use strategies and how they modify and interpret their use. Over time teachers will build up a body of knowledge about strategy use that they can use to troubleshoot individual problems and to enrich instruction.

Use the workshop sheets in the appendix to guide classroom instruction. Teachers can use part of the sheet to deliver a ten-minute lesson or to dedicate a whole class to strategy use. The sheets can also be used as handouts for self-study. It is important, however, to incorporate strategy use into skill development. Strategy use should not be developed in isolation from the contexts in which it is to be used. Students need to see strategy use as a tool for learning 'something.'

Take time to develop competent and routine strategy use. Strategy use takes years to master. Although students can enjoy the benefits of strategy use almost immediately, routine and competent use of learning strategies is a lifelong process. Even though I wrote the book on strategy use I still consider myself a 'learner.' I am constantly paying

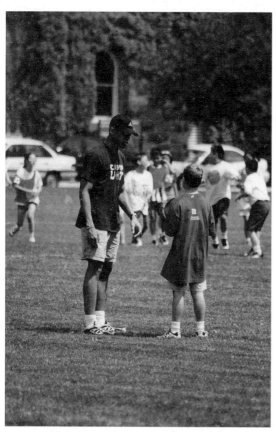

Reinforce the use of strategies.

attention to the strategy - its form, its application, and different ways to blend and combine the strategies. I am also amazed at how each person's perception of each strategy differs. Getting to know what sense students and teachers make of strategy use can be the subject of practice based research. Most of all, have fun with the strategies. They are tools designed to enrich the learning process and the attention students pay to their own thinking and the way they practice.

Building Understanding

♦ Prepare an explanation for parents that explains why learning strategies should be included in the physical education program.

Discuss the following with a partner:

♦ Of what benefit are learning strategies to learners? To teachers?

♦ Why should strategy use be an integral part of the physical education program?

♦ Compose a story that you could tell students about learning a skill that would convince them that strategically thinking about what you are doing is an important part of learning.

♦ How might the use of learning strategies in class affect the way you present concepts and skills, practice, give feedback, and evaluate achievement?

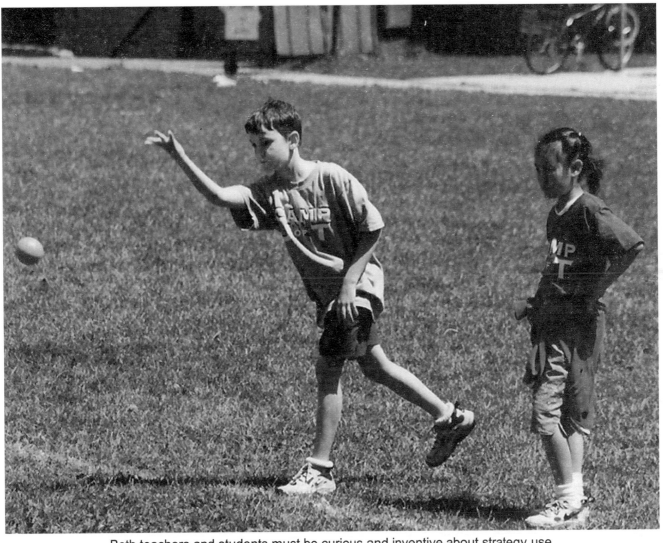

Both teachers and students must be curious and inventive about strategy use.

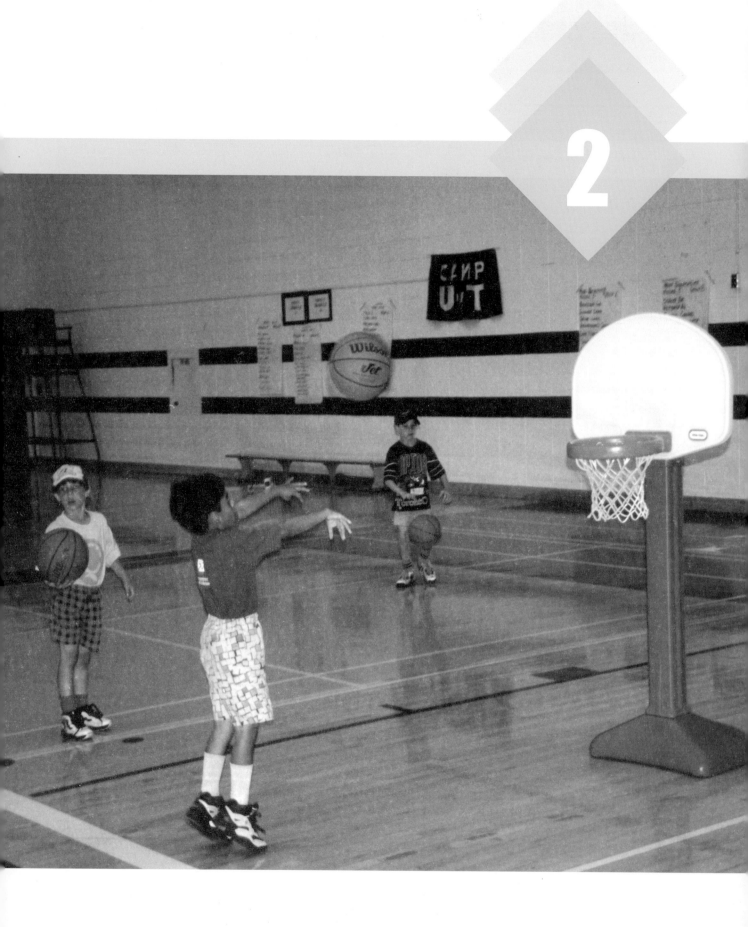

2

LEARNING STRATEGIES

Chapter Objectives

Define learning strategies

Recognize importance of strategy use

Relate strategy use to learning and skill improvement

Relate strategy use to healthy active living

Consider ways strategy use can become an integral part of instruction

Learning strategies are the cognitive tools used to systematically manage the thought processes associated with knowledge and skill acquisition (Anderson, 1992).

Everyone uses an assortment of strategies to remember information, concentrate on important tasks, and plan progress towards a goal. A window washer who came to your door

offering to clean your windows at a special rate, might ask how many windows you have in your home. How would you figure out mentally how many windows might require cleaning? Would you visualize each room and the number of windows? Parallel parking is another common situation in which self-talk and imagery may be used spontaneously. I often listen to drivers talk themselves through the process, cautioning, cueing and evaluating the performance as it unfolds: "Easy does it; yes, just a bit further; straighten out those wheels; hey, not bad."

We make plans every day. We anticipate our work schedule, leisure time, appointments, and household duties, and in response to the demands of each task, we budget time and resources accordingly. Mental imagery and self-talk are effective ways to think through, anticipate, and plan solutions to problems. Capable learners use these and a variety of other effective strategies with proficiency and regularity. The information about strategies presented here is aimed at providing teachers and students with descriptions and activities that can be a part of the formal instruction needed for routine and systematic use. Incorporating learning strategies into the learning process should reduce the number of errors and increase the number of successful trials, ensuring advancement to a more mature, controlled movement pattern in less time and with much less anxiety (Anderson, 1992).

Strategy use has been an important part of high-performance athletic activity. The psychology of sport has become an important interdisciplinary study merging sport science and psychology. It is common for athletes to use self-talk (Landin, 1994), imagery (Hall, Martin, Moritz, & Vadocz, 1995; Orlick, 1986), and goal-setting (Burton, 1992) as an integral part of the training process. Strategy use, practiced routinely and monitored by both the athlete and the coach (or sport psychologist), helps participants to cope with the stresses of performance.

Leaving learning to chance is risky. On the other hand, providing learners with the intellectual tools required to be successful reduces the need for luck or divine intervention. It also tells learners that their own effort, persistence, and dedication are paying off. Many different types of strategies are suited for learning in physical education settings. Some strategies such as picture words help learners relate prior knowledge and experience to more complex movement forms, channel the learner's attention towards the key elements of performance or block distractions, while other strategies such as goal-setting help learners focus and direct attention (Williams, & Leffingwell, 1997; Anderson, 1992; Singer, 1986). Some strategies are performed mentally, such as imagery, while others, such as goal-setting, involve record keeping and detailed prescriptions. Regardless of the type, strategies prepare learners to become active, creative agents of their own learning.

Two stories in the boxed sections illustrate the importance of being able to think both contextually and strategically and can be shared with students and parents. In the first story, you will read about what happens when participants are dependent on others to do the thinking. In the second story, Gina is talking to herself, but her 'inner voice' is not helpful; in fact, it adds to her anxiety.

There are several questions physical educators must consider. If we want to empower students to think for themselves, what tools are needed? How can teachers prepare students like Gina to not only hit the ball, but also cope with the distractions and tensions associated with athletic performance? Do teacher demonstrations and explanations adequately prepare students to hit the ball in situations where they are nervous or self-conscious? What would enable Gina to do what she wants to do, despite interferences? In addition to teaching students how to move, should physical educators also teach students how to think about their movements?

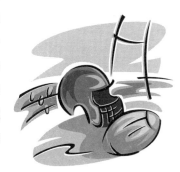

Ernie's Story

During a 1924 high school football game, Ernie Seiler, coach of Miami High, wanted to give quarterback Froggy Buchannan help calling the plays. Seiler lined up three water buckets on the sideline and kicked over the appropriate one to indicate run, pass, or punt. With Miami on the opponents' 18-yard line, Seiler accidentally kicked over the wrong bucket. Without thinking, Froggy punted the ball out of the end zone and into a store across the street. The annals of sport history are full of anecdotes such as the one above, where athletes have performed unwittingly and where blind obedience to the directions of the coaches have cost them more than just a victory.

Gina's Story

The bases are loaded. There's two out. I'm up to bat. I know I've just gotta hit that ball. The first ball comes to me. Easy. Easy. Looks good. I swing. The teacher yells out emphatically, "STRIKE ONE." Okay Gina, just wait. Take it easy. You don't have to swing. Maybe you could draw a walk to first base. Yeah, that could work. Here comes the ball. A little low, but I can hit it. I swing. "STRIKE TWO."

My heart is beating faster. "We want a batter!" someone yells out. "C'mon Gina." My hands are getting sweaty. I tighten my grip and do a practice swing and then tap the bat on home plate for good luck. Please God, help me hit the ball. Here it comes. Looks good. I swing. "STRIKE THREE! YOU'RE OUT!" My heart sinks. I knew I couldn't do it. Why was I pretending?

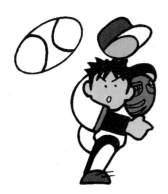

How Learning Strategies Work

Learning strategies prepare students to act with intention, focus, and diligence (Armstrong, Sallis, Hovell, & Hofstetter, 1993; Marcus, Selby, Niaura, & Rossi, 1992). According to Sage (1984), "the learning of a skill does not begin when actual practice starts, but before, with a cognitive understanding of the motor task" (p. 377). Before learners can attempt a task they must acquire some sense of what the task entails (i.e., the goal of the task, the movements needed to accomplish the goal, and the strategy necessary to generate the movements required). The sense (the looks/feels/sounds) that a person makes of the movement is described in the research literature as a cognitive map, cognitive plan, cognitive model, or template (Sage, 1984).

Map-making, when it pertains to movement, involves making connections between new actions and what is already known. In order for this to occur, each learner must actively engage in the construction of a motor plan (what am I expected to do? how will I position my body and limbs to achieve this outcome?). Learning is a deliberate process, a process that involves the learner assuming control over the action. Fortunately, learning strategies are tools that can be taught and managed by the students themselves to create links between what they already know and the task at hand.

A Closer Look at the Learning Process

The belief that learners interact and elaborate on their experiences has prompted both researchers and practitioners to pay closer attention to the ways learners consider and make sense of instruction.

Cognitive processing activities heighten the learner's awareness of the key features of the task, how the body actions relate to other movement concepts or experiences (e.g., does the underhand arm action look like an elephant swinging its trunk back and forth?).

Affective processing activities are concerned with the emotions involved in learning. Think back to Gina's story. Worrying about whether she would hit the ball interfered with her ability to concentrate on what to do to hit the ball. Throughout the learning process students will experience cycles of 'hot' and 'cold.' Hot periods occur when the learner is interested, focused, and persistent. Cold periods occur when the learner is out of touch with what is going on. Whether a participant is 'hot' or 'cold' may be dependent on a number of factors: amount of rest, nutrition, perceived importance of the task, etc. To increase engagement, educators need to heighten the participant's involvement in the activity, as well as the sense of mental and physical control required.

Metacognitive processing activities involve learners in making a conscious effort to be aware of their thinking and the actions that occur as a result of that thinking with respect to predetermined goals. Competent learners plan, monitor, test, and evaluate their work.

Cognitive Processing Activities:

♦**Structuring:** Is this a throwing movement?

♦**Relating:** Does this action (or part of it) look like any other movements I know?

♦**Analyzing:** How does the movement start/finish/produce force?

♦**Applying:** In what situations (playground games, athletic competition) could this skill be used?

Affective Processing Activities:

♦**Attributing:** I have a strong picture of the movement pattern.

♦**Motivating:** This is a skill I really want to learn.

♦**Concentrating:** I feel confident about my ability to focus on the key parts of the skill.

♦**Making judgments:** I like the way I did that.

♦**Appraising:** What parts do I need to improve? What did I leave out?

♦**Exerting effort:** I will try harder.

♦**Expecting:** If I concentrate on the 'right' things, I know I can accomplish my goals.

Metacognitive Processing Activities:

♦**Orienting:** Am I aware of the key features of the task?

♦**Planning:** What is my plan of action based on the information provided?

♦**Monitoring:** How will I keep track of my progress?

♦**Testing:** Can I apply the skill or knowledge to real-life situations in and outside school?

♦**Diagnosing:** Can I recognize errors?

♦**Evaluating:** How do my results compare with the expectations?

♦**Reflecting:** What kind of thinking works for me? What strategies work for me?

Beliefs About Learning That Support Strategy Use

Learning strategy use is based on the belief that learning is an interactive, sense-making process. Learning is interactive in that new ideas shape, and are, in turn, shaped by, existing ideas, beliefs, and understandings (Jones, Palinscar, Ogle, & Carr, 1987). New ideas shape or reshape the way people think and do things. For example, beginning golfers are more concerned about hitting the ball hard than hitting it well. Presented with information about how to hit properly, and the fact that hitting well translates into hitting straight and further, they may alter their views and work on achieving a more technically proficient swing. In many instances we may need to determine the initial beliefs of the learners. Some beliefs may be inaccurate and learners may have to rethink about performance and outcome achievement.

Existing ideas shape new ideas in that they are part of the way new ideas are interpreted. The beginning golfer, intent on developing a powerful swing, may selectively attend to information that, it is believed, will enhance his/her ability to hit the ball hard (e.g., an exaggerated over-rotated back-swing, tensing of the muscles during downswing and upon ball contact). Preconceived ideas about hitting the ball hard may interfere or divert attention away from details that would eventually enable the golfer to hit the ball better, further, consistently, and accurately.

The story about my nephew (see box) illustrates the power preconceived ideas can have on learning a new skill.

Interaction Between Existing and New Ideas

A two-way interchange of ideas is the key to understanding and thus has implications for instruction. The instructor must determine what ideas learners have already constructed about the task to be learned (what beliefs do the learners have about the skill that are counterproductive or useful?). In some instances, it may then be necessary to convince learners that their beliefs are either incomplete, inappropriate, or erroneous.

Existing Ideas

New Information

Remember the beginner golfer? It is critical that the beginner understand that hitting well is more productive than hitting hard.

Beginning with the learner's existing beliefs and understanding respects the learner as an active partner. When we understand the learner's reasoning we can begin to understand the learner's motives, which enables instruction to be tailored to the learner's particular interests and needs. The golfer might be more apt to listen and respond to instruction if the information relates specifically to the factors that influence the distance a ball travels and what influences the flight pattern of the ball. Simply giving instructions related to mechanics may not enable the learner to connect the instructional information to the golfer's agenda. Gearing instruction to the learner means finding out what type of learners (visual, kinesthetic, auditory) they are - their fears, goals, and reasons for learning the skill - and then finding ways to accommodate, alter, and enrich those beliefs. Existing ideas tell the teacher what the learners may already understand and what they need to understand in order to improve their skills.

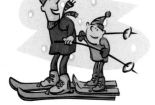

The interaction between existing and new ideas can also be an ef-

A Novice Skier

My 12-year-old nephew was invited to ski with our family. This was the first time he had ever skied. As we rode up the chairlift he remarked how closely some of the turning movements resembled ice skating. Although I pointed out that we were going to start with some other skills first, it was apparent to me that, in his mind, skiing and skating were similar and he believed that if he could skate, he could ski. As soon as we got off the chairlift he looked down the hill and proceeded to try out his theory. Until he worked out his own ideas about skiing he was not ready for my instruction. I waited and listened to the questions he asked to determine what he needed to know. When he was ready for instruction I began by building on his beliefs. "You sound like you are interested in learning to turn. You're right, hockey stops and turning are related. Show me what you do when you go into a hockey stop. What did you do with your legs? Right, you bent them as you turned your hips. Let's ski to the right and do just one hockey stop. Start tall and bend your knees into the turn. Keep your feet shoulder-width apart. Think of your skis as really long ice skates."

ficient and effective way of developing understanding. Learning, as indicated earlier, is a sense-making process. The learner constructs personal versions of what is experienced or presented through instruction by interpreting new ideas relative to existing beliefs and experiences. Interpretation is enhanced and refined by two important activities or engines that enable the learner to understand and apply knowledge in practical situations. These engines are elaboration and integration.

Elaboration

Elaboration occurs when a learner deepens and intensifies the awareness of an experience. Elaboration can occur in several ways. One way learners elaborate on experience is by explaining (in their own words) what the experience means to them. Elaboration is an individual's way of connecting to information. Knowledge makes more sense when it is under-

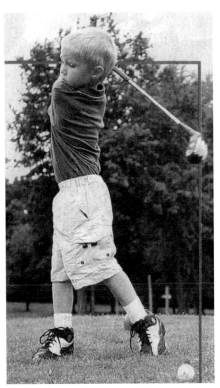

Strategy use sensationalizes experience.

stood subjectively, rather than objectively. When the Skydome was built in Toronto everyone had a different version of their first visit. Some marveled at the retractable roof, others thought the food vendors were terrific. Each person had a different story about the same building. Fishing expeditions are also highly vulnerable to elaboration. Elaboration involves adding flavour, character, and personal touches to an experience that enables the storyteller to remember and communicate details that might otherwise be forgotten.

Imagery and self-talk facilitate elaboration. Imagery involves forming mental representations that contain visual, kinesthetic, auditory, and gustatory details related to a physical performance. For imagery to be effective, the learner must first discover these details or become more aware of them. By attending closely to the pattern, the sound, and the feel of the action of the forehand tennis swing, the learner creates a mental template of the skill that is sensually more elaborate than if the learner simply observed the action. The imagery-educated learner sensationalizes experience creating a more intense

Learning strategy use teaches students that learning is:

♦ a conscious attempt to make sense of instruction and experience

♦ manageable: "I can control what I think and do"

♦ purposeful: goal-oriented

♦ manipulated to meet learner and content demands

♦ an active **process** that involves mind, body, and spirit

♦ about making connections

♦ different for each student

♦ dependent upon the learner's interpretation of what happens

♦ influenced by interest, curiosity, prior experience, and emotion

mind/body relationship with the skill and has a more sophisticated and personal understanding of the skill.

Self-talk is a script the learner co-creates about a skill. Self-talk that contains metaphors and analogies promotes personalization and connections between existing knowledge and the new material presented. The use of metaphoric self-talk for the arm action for the forehand tennis swing might be, "sweep the crumbs off the table." Using terms the learner already knows and has experienced in order to make sense of new ideas is a powerful way of absorbing and retaining information, and avoiding the cognitive overload common during the early stages of skill acquisition.

Integration

The second engine in the sense-making process is integration. Integration involves making the new information an integral part of thought and action. Students who know that swinging a golf club hard will not necessarily produce better results but continue to swing with all their strength, have not integrated the 'right' ideas about the golf swing. Some of the reasons learners fail to integrate are listed below.

1. New ideas may not be integrated because the existing knowledge is entrenched. Bad and old habits are difficult to change.

2. New ideas fail to provide an alternative that is compelling enough to alter existing attitudes. Learning to swing smoothly and in a relaxed manner may not appeal to golfers who view themselves as power hitters.

3. New ideas may not initially provide enough evidence to dislodge existing beliefs: "Why is this new method so much better? Even when I try to hit smoothly, the ball still slices."

4. New ideas may not have a significant impact on the learner: to be effective, the learner must interact with the content in ways that make sense to him/her. The learner must be equipped to engage actively in a process that relates means and ends in relation to personal goals, interests, and abilities.

Strategic Learners

In every class there will be individuals who, with limited instruction, know what to do. They may anticipate equipment and spatial needs, suggest alternative ways to perform a skill, work well with limited or no supervision, and acquire new skills and apply them well to varied and novel situations. These children display characteristics of the strategic learner. Put simply, the strategic learner, according to Beimiller and Meichenbaum (1992), knows what to do to be successful and does it without being told.

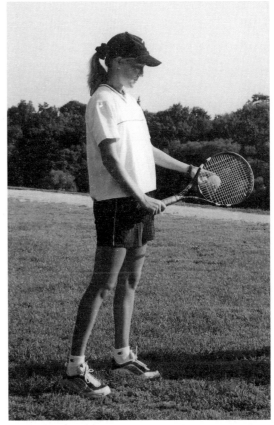

Strategic learners are thoughtful and planful.

Strategic learners monitor situations and tasks and respond accordingly. We might say, strategic learners have their act together (they coordinate thought and action). Successful players and teams execute a well-thought-out plan. Anyone who wants to become a better golfer knows s/he must understand course management. The approach to each green is surveyed in advance and a set of shots is carefully selected in relation to the terrain, hole placement, and any hazards that are placed along the fairway. Playing the course, not the other players, is what the strategists think about.

Strategic fishermen do not randomly select a location to fish. They have carefully mapped out the body of water they intend to fish according to its habitat (food, predators, protection) and characteristics (depth, water temperature, flow of water). In this way, the angler methodically calculates the potential each area has to yield particular kinds of fish. Cast patterns cross-section a target area maximizing opportunities to 'catch the big one.'

Physical education students who exhibit expert-like qualities are not ready to compete in the Olympics or play professional sport; however, they are mature in their skill understandings and behaviour, for their age and stage of development. How do children arrive at this level of insight and performance? What happened along the way that

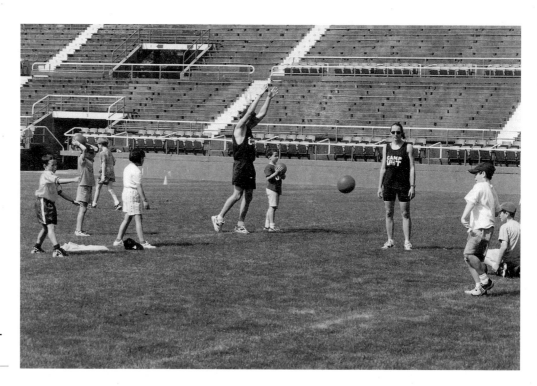

Incorporate strategy use throughout instruction and practice.

prompted these enviable qualities? Can teachers and parents reproduce the conditions that generate these outcomes? Throughout the literature, expert learners are commonly referred to as self-directed learners and are defined as individuals who can deal with problems on their own. Early research in self-directed learning stemmed from attempts to create artificial intelligence in computers. Studies of expertise in various aspects of human endeavour included professional athletics, chess, business, gardening, food service, engineering, and medicine.

The development of expertise in physical education classes involves the ability to intelligently manage a number of instructional resources in varied and often complex situations. Derry (1990) reminds us that successful academic learners have a range of strategies from which they are able to select and adapt to meet the needs of a specific situation. To become competent learners, students need to be aware of what they are doing, know how to monitor their actions, and know how to refine their errors (Weinstein & Mayer, 1986; Meichenbaum & Beimiller, 1990).

In addition to teaching students how to catch and throw properly, physical educators can teach children how to learn how to catch and throw. The quality of each practice trial and the rate of progress toward mastery both increase for those in control of the learning process. Teachers, too, feel good about enabling students to do more for themselves.

Links Between Strategy Use and Healthy Active Living

Learning strategies play an integral role in both the commitment and capacity to lead healthy active lives by facilitating both knowledge acquisition and knowledge application. Learning strategies provide learners with the tools necessary to build and make use of their knowledge in the pursuit of sport, recreation, and leisure activities.

Physically educated individuals know the value of strategy use and have a commitment and capacity to lead a healthy, active life. Capacity refers to the knowledge and skills needed to participate in a wide variety of physical activities. Capacity also refers to the ability to regulate physical, emotional, and cognitive involvement in task achievement (e.g., monitoring and reflecting on outcomes in relation to performance standards, personal goals, abilities, and interests).

Commitment refers to the individual's will to achieve. Learners who can focus on the means necessary for success rather than just the end result will use strategies to enhance performance and to treat mistakes as learning challenges. They will attribute success to personal effort and will persist despite the setbacks they encounter. The pursuit of any physical skill is dependent upon the learner's aspirations, goals, motives and strength of mind to maintain participation despite obstacles and challenges. Without commitment, the struggle to succeed may be short-lived and erratic. Learning strategies such as goal-setting help learners plot progress in ways that meet their present and emerging interests. Goals help learners systematically align their needs, interests, and ambitions. Goal-setting enables learners to clarify their motives for participation and to mobilize their efforts towards achieving their goals as active, healthy learners.

Factors Distinguishing Self-directed Learners:

♦ **Knowledge:** experts know more about a subject and have the information organized for rapid retrieval and efficient and effective use

♦ **Strategies:** experts have an assortment of cognitive tools that enable them to guide the thought processes that promote learning

♦ **Motivation:** experts go out of their way to acquire new knowledge and skills

Links Between Strategy Use and Active Learning

Active learning means that, as much as possible, learners are involved in manipulating content materials and ideas. In addition to performing mechanically correct movement patterns, learners are encouraged to understand how each movement pattern relates to game play in a variety of contexts, as well as how they relate to other skills within the physical education program.

For example, how does the overhand throwing pattern developed in grades one and two relate to throwing a football in grades four and five? How does knowledge of throwing transfer to serving in tennis or volleyball? In what other activities is the overhand throw a fundamental component?

Creating an environment that is conducive to active learning depends on the teacher's willingness and ability to:

a. understand the learner's perceptions of the situation or task

b. help learners connect with the content

c. elicit learner interest in the material

d. integrate information about motor learning and the mechanical aspects of a skill to create learning challenges that capture several key features together (for example, if learners are instructed to 'jump to the ball' as they attempt an instep soccer kick, hip flexion will occur automatically and the momentum of the action will produce follow through. There is no need to teach each element separately).

For learning to occur, students must think strategically about what they are doing, make decisions about the purpose of their actions, reflect on the quality of outcomes in relation to goals, and revise their performance according to their observations and evaluations.

Sage (1984) indicates that mental practice techniques are more efficient with beginners because cognitive aspects of the task are more salient at this stage. As learners attempt to construct an image of the goal, the task, and how to accomplish the task, they need to identify the key features of performance. He suggests strategy use has good potential for correcting errors in execution, increasing concentration, helping to gain perceptual insights, and assisting in strategy rehearsal.

Joint efforts by teachers and students to promote active learning through the use of learning strategies has several benefits. They are listed below.

A Better Understanding of the Task Demands

Imagery helps the learner structure the task using familiar images. Learners are encouraged to think about the task in ways that make sense to them (Meichenbaum, 1977). The identification and use of key images promotes more complete task comprehension and more frequent carryover use of the strategy in other situations.

Thoughtful Preparation and Execution of the Skill

Self-talk gives learners a chance to mentally rehearse or to recite movement sequences in advance (Shasby, 1986; Weiss & Klint, 1987). This makes each practice trial higher in quality.

Weiss and Klint (1987) studied the developmental differences between modeling and verbal rehearsal on the performance of a sequential motor task among two groups, aged five to six and eight to nine. They found that a visual model may not be a sufficient means of instruction. Verbal rehearsal strategies are also needed to help children selectively attend to relevant task components and to remember the specific order in which skills should be executed.

Transfer to Related Movement Challenges and to Direct Skill Acquisition in Novel Situations

For self-directed learners, learning strategies become a way of life. In other words, when faced with a movement challenge, proficient learners tend to find and use learning strategies that will help them meet the demands of the task.

Meichenbaum and Beimiller (1990) found that self-directed learners not only seem to have more information about assigned tasks, but they also reason with information sometimes modifying, substituting, or refining it on their own according to the context. Strategic

---

Active learning encourages students to:

♦ interpret experiences in relation to prior knowledge

♦ search for alternative perspectives and personal meaning

♦ reflect on outcomes in light of personal goals, purposes, and values. Accordingly, learners are expected to be pattern seekers, relationship finders, and problem solvers

knowledge appears to enable learners to work with minimal direction and prompting. Self-directed learners also appear to have higher levels of self-efficacy and expectations for success, which in turn influences task commitment and perseverance.

Heightened Awareness of the Need for and Impact of Learning Strategies   As students become more comfortable using learning strategies, they appreciate the great impact such strategies can have on their progress.

Regulated Learning   Through an enhanced capacity to monitor, analyze, and evaluate their own progress, self-directed learners are better able to think about their performances. Using what they already know about the task, they are able to reflect on the merits of their performance in relation to previously established criteria. Metacognitive processing activities, such as evaluating and reflecting, allow learners to learn from experience and trust the validity of their own insights. Strategic learners are more likely to learn from their mistakes as well as their successes and to attribute outcomes to their own efforts rather than to uncontrollable factors such as chance or innate ability (Vermunt, 1987).

Two-way Teaching   Listening to children's self-talk enables teachers to hear the mental operations governing learning behavior. When learners discuss their performance, contribute to a dialogue about the task, and make suggestions, teachers become co-investigators and facilitators.

Benefits of Learning Strategies

Learning Strategies:

- focus the learner's attention on relevant features of performance
- facilitate interaction between the learner and the content
- promote planning

- promote self-monitoring and self-evaluation
- promote insights into the learning process
- deepen the learner's understanding of the way s/he learns
- promote self-efficacy

Learning Strategies Summary

Learning strategies are the tools used to manage the thought processes associated with learning. When air conditioning was first introduced it was included in all luxury vehicles. Today air conditioning is standard equipment in almost all vehicles. Similarly, all learners, not just high performance athletes, can benefit from strategy use. Learning strategies enhance engagement (cognitive, affective, and physical) with learning experiences. Strategy users interact better with the content to make sense of the challenges before them. Strategic learners, like experts, approach learning purposefully and deliberately. Students involved in learning on their own are more likely to attribute success to their own efforts, try new skills, and overcome learning obstacles and disappointments. Strategic learners know they can control learning. Learning strategies empower students to do more for themselves.

Building Understanding

♦What do learners need to know about a skill (physically, mentally, and emotionally) to promote learning?

♦How can learners use learning strategies during the early stages of skill acquisition or during the application of skills to game situations to overcome self-doubt, anxiety, and fear of failure?

♦Based on what has been said here about the learning process, what changes do you think need to be made concerning your current teaching methods? What changes are necessary in the way students are expected to interact with each other and the content in class?

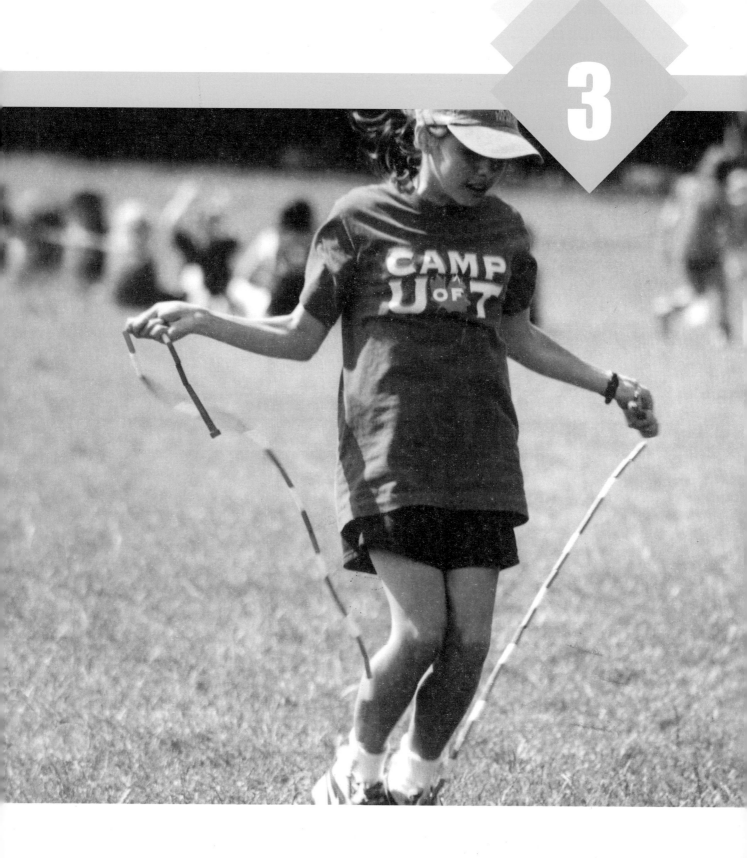

PICTURE WORDS

Chapter Objectives

Define picture words

Describe the benefits of picture word use

Relate picture word use to learning

Teach picture word use in physical education and coaching settings

Picture words add life to descriptions—they portray sensations and imagination.

Definition of Picture Words

Picture words are used to depict a specific action or skill. Self-directed learning begins with the use of picture words. Although picture words are initially selected by the teacher, their choice soon becomes the responsibility of the students themselves, and thus an integral part of translating information into self-instructional prompts or cues. Picture words introduce students to ways of thinking about body actions using relevant and familiar images. Children are already good at 'pretending,' 'make-believe,' and using their imaginations. Creating 'make-believe' situations involves many of the same cognitive activities children are expected to carry out when planning to perform fundamental motor tasks in class. If children can 'plot' a series of make-believe actions (pretending to be a firefighter or a teacher), it seems reasonable to apply this self-directing capacity to motor learning situations.

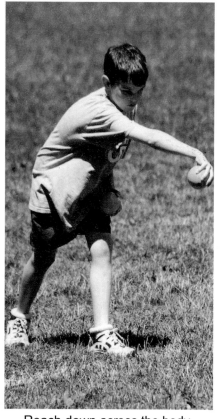

Reach down across the body.

Picture words, then, use metaphors, similes, and analogies to describe movement patterns ("swinging the elephant's trunk" to focus on the arm action for the underhand throw or using "McDonald's Golden Arch" to describe the flight pattern of a ball. Picture words have a mnemonic purpose; they conjure up images a learner can use to remember an action sequence or key elements of form and thus to monitor progress. Encouraging students to create and use picture words is a friendly way of getting them comfortable and confident about using non-technical, familiar terms to describe body actions. Eventually, students who are more comfortable about talking to themselves can become accomplished in using imagery in many different ways. I sometimes ask for specific kinds of picture words (for example, "action words" – dash, slide; or "feeling words" – soft, stiff). Helping learners recognize the importance of connecting picture words to skill development enables them to realize that learning is an active process over which they can exercise considerable control but also one which requires perseverance for success.

Kinds of Picture Words

Picture words prompt visual images, feelings, sounds, and smells that learners relate to specific body actions, events, or activities. Consider the following examples: "sweep the crumbs off the table," to describe a

Picture Words and Sensory Modalities

Seeing Words: help learners create visual images. For example, think or say aloud, "Open Batman's cape," to remember to hold your arms out at your sides for balance before you approach the in-step soccer kick.

Hearing Words: help learners connect to the sound of the movement. For example, think or say, "punch" when you finish a round-off to increase height when you rebound off the floor.

Feeling Words: can evoke strong physical and emotional responses. For example, keep the picture word, "glide" in your mind as you swing your arms when you cross- country ski.

forehand tennis swing; "throw your hands at the ball," to promote batting accuracy; "cradle the ball" to encourage retraction of the arms when catching a football. These picture word phrases can be used by youngsters to acquire and refine movement patterns with confidence. Students can use these phrases independently and also use them to help their friends improve their own skills. They can also become adept at error detection and provide corrective feedback to themselves and others.

Some picture words direct a learner's attention to performance outcomes, influencing the force, tempo, or pace of the action. Words like "explode," "rocket ship," and "burst" produce stronger and quicker actions. Some words like "float" and "melt" can trigger a more fluid motion. In these instances, an attempt is made to control effort and focus on proficiency and efficiency.

Other picture words are used to alleviate tension and anxiety. Picture words such as "marshmallows," "feathers," "trickle," or "pillow" help the learner 'soften' both the body and the mind. This is important for activities such as catching. Catching skills are much harder to perform if the arms and hands are kept rigid. When learning to catch, learners can pretend their hands are spider webs, trying not to break the spider web strands as they catch the bean bag. They may also try to pretend the bean bag is landing on marshmallows or a pillow to make a soft landing. These cues will help arms naturally contract or 'give' into the body.

The ability to relax is a life skill that can be learned in physical education and applied to stressful situations. For example, relaxation skills can be used to prepare to give a speech, take a driver's test, prepare or recover from surgery, control anger, or hit a ball when friends are watching. Picture words can also be used in other classes as a means of stress management (e.g., what word might help you relax when you are really stressed out: "feathers," "whipped cream"?). A single relaxing word can be connected to a larger script. For example, students might listen to a description of a tropical beach. After several minutes of listening and thinking about the sights, sounds, and smells associated with the beach, students are reminded they can return to the scenes and experiences they created any time by simply saying the word "beach."

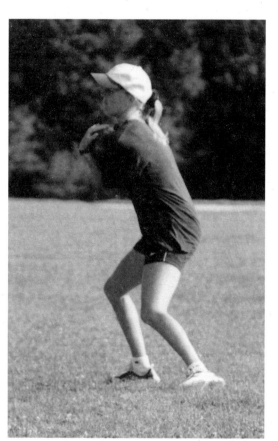

Get behind and below the ball.

Similarly, students working on the overhand throw have viewed and prepared a script for specific body movements. For example, the basic overhand throw can be portrayed as, "stand sideways," "spread the wings of the eagle" (to show the arms extended in preparation for the throw), "twist out from underneath the throw" (to show hip rotation), and "scratch the knee" (to show follow-through with the throwing arm down and across the body). Before students execute the throw, they must pause and momentarily imagine themselves performing the skill. Trigger words, such as "wings," "twist out," and "scratch" form an action phrase that enables students to refocus mentally on the key elements of performance prior to performance. It is best to limit the number of picture words in an action phrase to three to five words. As students master elements of form, picture words can be dropped from the action phrase.

How Picture Words Work

Knowledge is not stored in isolated bits but is encoded into schematic networks. For example, a simple experience such as jumping into a pool of water, generates a whole range of information that goes beyond the action itself. We absorb aspects about the sensation of flight prior to immersion, the sounds and feelings of splashing, the first contact with the water temperature, the feelings of immersion, submersion, and ascent to the surface—in addition to the joy or fear that may surround the event. The array of mental constructs generated by the total experience becomes a knowledge base upon which other actions and emotions can be associated. These existing competencies are a resource used to make sense of new experiences. Picture words provide powerful mnemonic tools especially when two properties exist: associability - concepts and words are imaginable and meaningful; and constructability - they can be recalled reliably from memory on different occasions to produce the results intended. Years after teaching a group of third graders how to throw using picture words and self-talk, they still recall "spread the wings of the eagle," "twist out," and "scratch."

Benefits of Picture Word Use

Teaching students how to use picture words enables them to work independently and methodically, recall more information, detect errors, and remain focused on a task for longer periods of time. Picture words can also be taught to both young and old. Picture words used to learn a basic

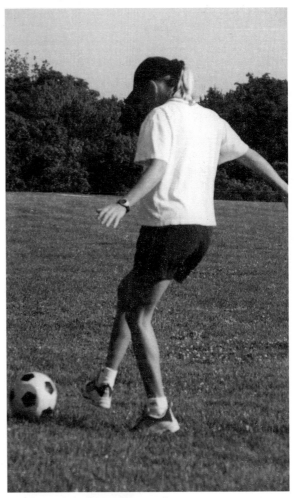

Open Batman's cape.

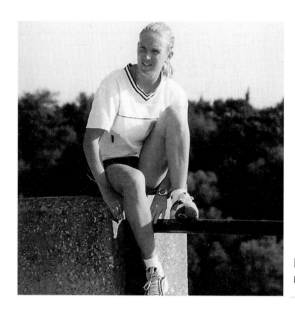

Picture words help people remember what to do.

skill can be transferred to related and more difficult skills. For example, the underhand throw descriptors ("swing the elephant's trunk") can be applied to underhand throws using a plastic scoop and the underhand serve in volleyball. Learners with perceptual motor difficulties may also benefit from the use of picture words to help remember and guide performance. The more students remember, the more confident and focused they will be during practice.

According to Gordon (1961), metaphors and analogies foster involvement, because the learner is able to interact with the content in a more personable way; detachment, which enables the learner to stand

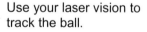

Use your laser vision to track the ball.

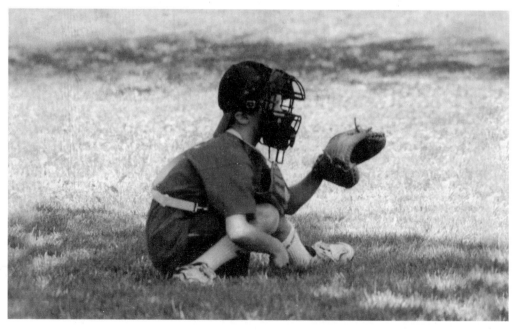

back and view situations, tasks, and experiences objectively; deferment, which allows the learner to set aside or stand away from problems until the best solution is reached; speculation, which allows the mind to roam free so it can come up with ideas; and autonomy of object, because the use of metaphors and analogies moves the learner from the immediacy of "I" to the symbolic, reflective, contemplative position of "me."

Benefits of using picture words:

♦ remember what to do

♦ focus on quality actions

♦ connect existing knowledge and experience to new learning

♦ promote self-directed learning

Psychoanalysts suggest that self-observation works at the interface of I and me permitting and encouraging exploration and analysis at three levels:

♦ **immediate awareness:** what I saw, felt, heard, experienced

♦ **mediated awareness:** what happened to me, what the experience meant to me

♦ **dynamic awareness:** the on-going relationship between the two

Picture Words and Self-regulated Learning

Picture words provide a cognitive link between existing knowledge, skills, and movement images and what is to be learned. Relation to content affects a student's ability to control thought and action. Picture words draw learners mentally closer to the actions they perceive as

The use of picture words, feeling words, and hearing words introduces students to the idea that:

♦ everyday language, terms, and experiences can be used to make sense of new content

♦ picture words help people remember what to do

♦ picture words are portable - that is, learners can carry instructional information with them between school and home to help practice skills

♦ personal descriptions (meanings) count as long as they accurately depict the outcomes desired

relevant. The more control learners exert over their actions, the more likely they will be able to regulate their performance—that is, plan ahead, make changes, evaluate outcomes, and set targets on their own.

Links Between Picture Word Use and Peer Learning

The use of picture words encourages learners to assess their own performances and those of their peers. In peer learning situations, students are paired to help each other create and use picture words to enhance their progress. Peer learning strategies enable students to work collaboratively with instructional materials to improve their skills (see Chapter 7). This takes time and trust. Initially, students are hesitant to give their peers instruction. Teachers must model and encourage peer teaching, inviting students to "be the teacher," and use the picture words to give feedback during simulation demonstrations. Reinforcing the constructive nature of peer work will help students overcome reluctance to give advice or to accept criticism.

Picture word use facilitates interaction between different age groups. Older students can work with younger students because the language is friendly and familiar, yet informative. Just as reading buddies and writing buddies help students develop language skills, physical education buddies can be used to promote skill development.

A Three-phased Approach to Picture Word Use

There are three phases to the use of picture words. Each phase is distinguished by a particular teacher-student-content relationship.

Phase One is largely teacher-directed. Students are dependent on the teacher to invent and supply the terms used to describe the body action. Selection and depiction are induced by the teacher. For example, to instruct the basic overhand throw the teacher might use the following picture words:

Phase One

It is the teacher's responsibility to:

- demonstrate the outcomes expected (usually elements of form, behaviour, pattern, etc.)
- identify the key elements of performance students are expected to achieve, reviewing in advance what you will accept as evidence of achievement and remembering only to focus on one or two elements of form at a time
- select terms that are friendly – terms that students readily connect with
- give feedback using the picture, feeling, and hearing words presented in class (e.g., "Remember to spread those wings"; "You did a nice job making the catch quiet")
- assess student progress relative to the key elements discussed in class
- report this progress to students and to parents using the terms adopted to describe skill achievement (e.g., "John's use of picture words has improved his throwing skills. He is able to demonstrate the proper throwing action consistently")
- check for accuracy to ensure proper form is habituated

It is the student's responsibility to:

- use picture words to describe the body actions
- assess his/her achievement and progress in relation to the picture words presented by the teacher
- observe and judge other performances in relation to class discussion and instruction

- *"stand sideways"*
- *"spread the wings of the eagle"*
- *"BIG 'J'"*
- *"step over the line"*
- *"twist your hips out from underneath you"* or *"naval attack"*
- *"throw"*
- *"scratch"*

Phase Two

It is the teacher's responsibility to:

♦provide a quality demonstration of the outcomes expected

♦identify the key elements of performance

♦encourage students to select picture, feeling, and hearing words to describe the body action

♦provide feedback to students in relation to their use of the picture words for self-guidance

♦assess achievement of the key elements of performance

♦ monitor the use of picture words

♦report to students and parents about the key elements of performance (e.g., "Josie selects good picture words to guide her thinking about the instep kick")

It is the student's responsibility to:

♦cooperate creatively with the teacher in devising picture words used to describe the body actions expected

♦use these picture words to guide instruction

♦use these picture words to detect and correct errors

♦use the terms to assess his/her own progress

♦use the terms to assess the achievement of peers

Phase Two encourages students to participate in the construction and selection of picture words to describe the body action. For example, after demonstrating how to trap a soccer ball, a teacher may invite students to substitute picture, feeling, and hearing words for the action. The teacher's explanation might be: "Using the instep part of the foot, draw it back as contact is made so the ball won't bounce off the foot." Encouraged to create their own picture words, students might respond: "Use the big foot (wide part of foot) to make a quiet, soft stop like it hit a pillow."

Phase Three allows the learner to move a step closer to self-directed learning. Students are shown the movement but the explanations and key elements of form are identified largely by the student. The teacher may need to coach the selection somewhat, but with little or no prompting the students will choose picture words that contain appropriate images, feelings, and sounds for the action.

Over time students build up a movement vocabulary. In movement journals students may compile their list of action words, special terms, or develop a movement dictionary that contains illustrations and descriptions of key body actions.

Creating an Illustrated Picture Word Dictionary

A great way of integrating the power of language with the development of movement concepts is to list action words and have students illustrate each one. The results can be displayed in both the gymnasium and the classroom. Some students may even choose to be more creative by developing wire sculptures or plasticine figures to illustrate specific movements.

Phase Three

It is the teacher's responsibility to:

- demonstrate contrasting examples of the skill or behaviour
- display their inferences
- encourage students to label or name the key features of the skill or action
- encourage students to use the terms they select to guide their practice
- assess abilities to identify movement patterns presented in the demonstrations (e.g., "Maya can identify the key body actions for basic skills such as underhand catching and throwing and select appropriate picture words to describe the key features")

It is the student's responsibility to:

- look for connections between the skill and familiar actions and images
- select and use picture, feeling, and hearing words to describe the body action
- share picture words with the rest of the class to build up a movement vocabulary, with the aim eventually of keeping a movement journal, containing illustrations and descriptions of key body actions

Examples of Action Words

Locomotion	*Stability*	*Manipulation*
skate	tripod	juggle
skateboard	pretzel	hoola hoop

Handouts and Workshop Activities for Students

The picture words newsletter in the Appendix can be distributed to the students or displayed on a bulletin board. It can be used to promote discussion about the use of picture words or as part of a lesson that demonstrates the connection between picture words and body actions. For instance, give the students a picture word sequence such as: curl, stretch, melt; dash, freeze, squeeze; waddle, pounce, wriggle; crawl, crumple, fold. Discuss with students how picture words provide important ways of understanding movement, shape and size, and the distinct shape of

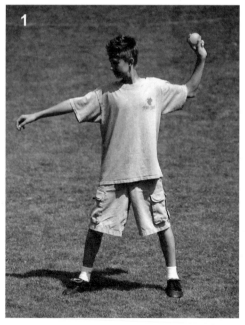

Stand sideways—"BIG 'J'."

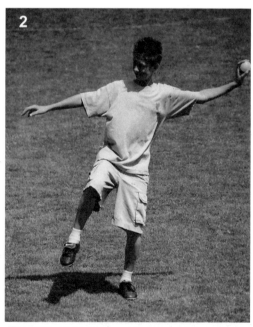

Spread the wings of the eagle. Rock back.

The teacher should make a list of picture words and display them under headings such as:

travelling	non-travelling	sinking	rising	stopping
gallop	*explode*	*deflate*	*grow*	*anchor*
————	————	————	————	————
————	————	————	————	————

an action or skill.

Have fun creating picture word phrases that can be displayed on large flash cards. For example, grow—spin—deflate; jump—freeze—jab; creep—pounce—explode (see Docherty, 1975).

Encourage students to create picture word phrases or action stories that depict for example, building a snowman, burying a treasure, barbecuing hotdogs, or shopping for groceries. These movement 'stories' can be recalled later to create imagery and self-talk scripts .

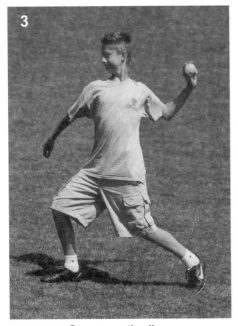

Step over the line.

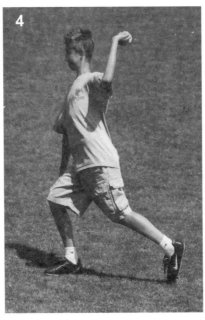

Twist your hips out from underneath you.

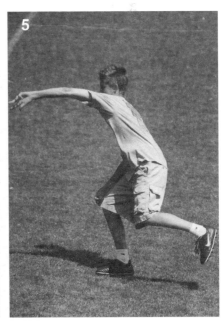

Throw.

Imagine you are going up to bat, to get into your batting stance...

Now, imagine starting to swing at the ball...

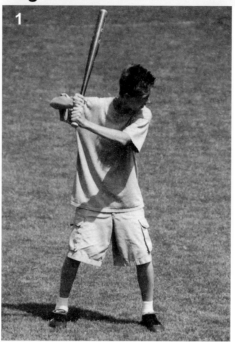

Pretend to throw a can of pop over your shoulder with your left hand. Place the other hand (right) on top of the left hand.

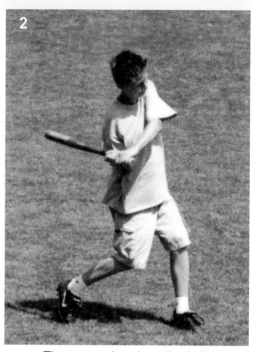

Throw your hands at the ball.

Picture Words Summary

Picture words enable the learner to relate familiar concepts and experiences to the movements they are learning. Picture words make learning 'friendly' and inviting. Picture words provide visual, kinesthetic, and auditory cues. Used properly, picture words enable the person to overcome many learning barriers. Instruction that includes the use of picture words is more likely to be remembered and used by the learners on their own, to reinforce key elements of performance, and to enhance focus.

… make contact…   **… and complete your swing!**

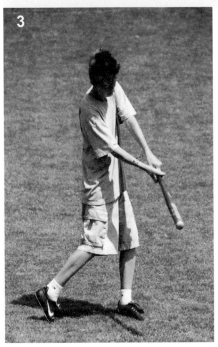

Squash the bug (twist out) with your foot.

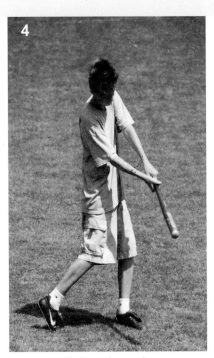

Follow through.

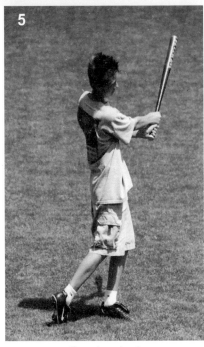

Good swing!

Building Understanding

♦ Why is it important to help students connect the use of picture words to physical skill development?

♦ What messages do teachers communicate to students about skill development through the use of picture words?

♦ What do teachers need to know about the mechanics of a skill in order to select and endorse the selection of picture words?

♦ At what age can teachers and coaches begin to use picture words to prompt actions?

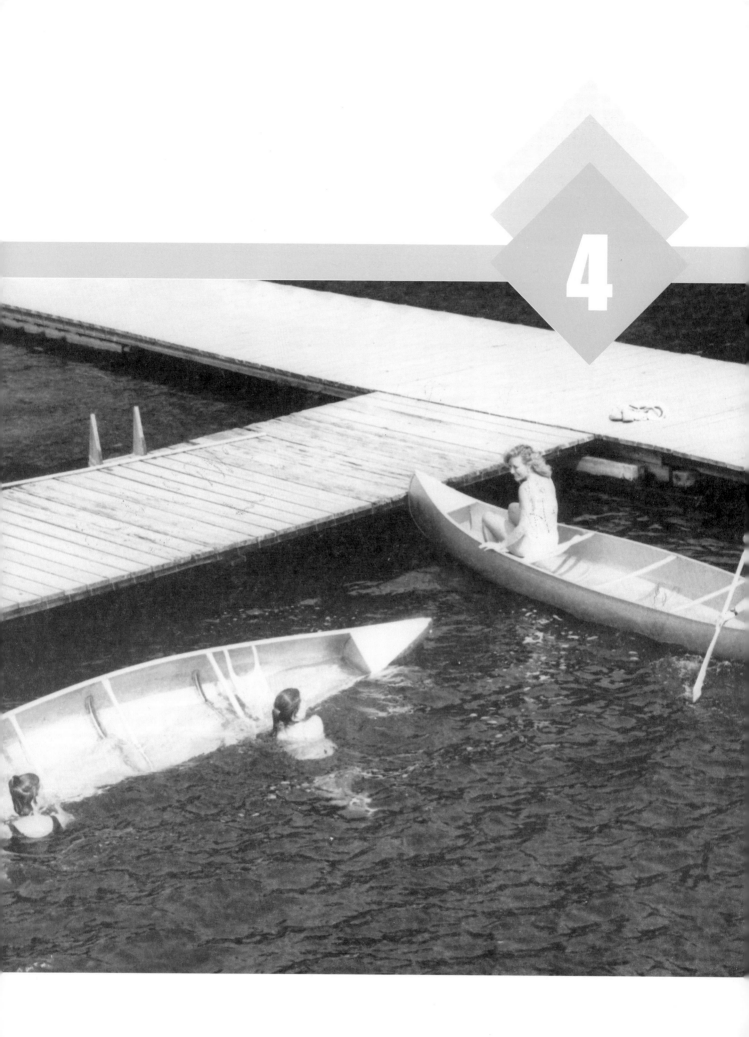

4

IMAGERY

Chapter Objectives

Define imagery

Distinguish different kinds of imagery

Describe the benefits of imagery use

Relate imagery use to sport performance

Relate imagery use to learning in physical education

Teach imagery use

Use classroom ready materials to build skills for imagery and self-reliant learning

Imagery sensationalizes learning—it enhances our sense of touch, sight, sound, and taste.

Definition of Imagery

Imagery is "the deliberate use of the senses to mentally rehearse a particular motor skill or movement sequence in the absence of, or in combination with overt physical movement" (Afremow, Overby, & Vadocz, 1996). Every day we hear how imagery has in some way influenced a person's thinking. Tell-tale phrases include: "I could never see myself doing that." "Picture that!" "In my mind's eye, this is how I pictured it would be." "I just had a mental picture of what that would be like." When words are not enough, or in some instances too much, we might use images (icons, symbols, graphic designs) to represent the important messages we want to remember. Images of war, poverty, violence, love, and compassion can have an enduring impact on our lives and convey a powerful message. We often say, "a picture is worth a thousand words."

Imagery is a trial run in our heads that awakens us physically, emotionally, and psychologically to a specific task.

Students studying for exams, for example, often develop notes that contain what may look like hieroglyphics. These specially coded messages render complex information and abstract ideas in a form the learner can assimilate cogently and easily. Images and symbols pervade everyday life, from traffic signs and warning labels, to computer desktops. Corporate logos are recognized around the world. At the age of two my daughter could identify the McDonald's golden arches as a place to eat and get a treat-of-the-week long before she could read. The Red Cross is recognized and respected globally as a symbol for medical care and disaster relief.

Imagery and daydreaming are different but related concepts. Imagery goes further than daydreaming in that it is a conscious, carefully constructed (re)enactment of an experience or performance we are planning to execute. Imagery is a mental trial run that awakens us physically, emotionally, and psychologically to a specific task. Imagery is consciously controlled, even scripted, to portray ourselves in our mind's eye in a certain way, in real time, in a particular context, helping us cope with obstacles and unforeseen challenges, and helping us achieve our goals. Daydreams, on the other hand, tend to be random mental wanderings.

It is not uncommon to daydream about athletic performance. I used to have this exciting daydream about being a goalie in the NHL. What was so thrilling about the daydream was that I saw all the action in slow motion. No matter how skilled the players were and how fast the puck was travelling, I could see the puck approaching at half the normal speed and, as a result, make the most spectacular saves. Mark Tewkesbury (Canada's 1992 Olympic Gold Medal winner in swimming) recalled his daydreams prior to his record breaking achievements at the Olympics. He said that for some time, when he daydreamed about himself on the podium after a competition, he could only see himself on the second and third place platforms. It wasn't until he was able to see himself standing on the first place platform during these daydream experiences that he realized he really could achieve a gold medal.

Our images of ourselves, then, have an impact on our performance. I remember asking children in grade two, "What does a physically fit person look like to you?" The girls' image of female fitness was "skinny"; the boys' image of male fitness was "big muscles." When asked, most students identified their mothers as those who exercised in the home. The women went to the 'Y,' followed an exercise program on television, or went to an exercise or health club, in order to lose weight or to be healthy. Interested about why fathers were not portrayed similarly, I asked, "Don't your fathers do anything for exercise—for example, play sports?" "Oh sure, they play sports," they replied, identifying a wide range of sports their fathers enjoyed: golf, hockey, slow pitch, etc. It seemed, however, that the children did not associate participation in sports with health and exercise. Exercise is what their mothers did as a choreographed activity to manage weight. Dads played sports to compete or to enjoy a night out with the boys. This example should help us recognize that images of exercise and sport may have an impact on the activity a student selects or a program in which he/she chooses to enroll.

Not having experienced something directly does not preclude imagining it. Although many of us may never have bungee jumped, we can nevertheless draw on an extensive range of experiences to imagine what a free fall might be like. At an early age many of us were tossed into the air and caught by our parents. Television also provides us with sensational close-ups of experiences such as bungee jumping. Microphones and cameras attached to participants allow us to make the jump vicariously, feeling the exhilaration of taking the plunge.

Perspectives in Imagery

Individually and collectively, mental images create powerful mental representations of real action that enable the person to be in the middle of the action, 'living' the event without actually performing it.

Stimulus-laden compositions contain imagery that may be sensitive to the environment or to situational demands. Put plainly, you are acutely aware of what is going on around you. Murphy and Jowdy (1992) provide a script that illustrates the characteristics of stimulus compositions:

> You are engaged in a training run down a street close to your home on a beautiful autumn day. You are wearing a bright red track suit; and as you run, you watch the wind blowing the leaves from the street onto the neighbor's lawn. A girl on a bicycle passes you, and you see that she is delivering newspapers. You swerve to avoid a pothole in the road, and you smile at another runner passing you in the opposite direction.

In this example, the runner is not paying much attention to body actions and how his/her movements respond to the environment. The runner is aware of what objects are around but not his/her reaction or feelings in relation to these objects/events.

Response-laden compositions contain images focused on the individual's response to situations and tasks. Murphy and Jowdy (1992) provide another illustration:

Kinds of Imagery

♦**Visual:** picturing the activity or event in your mind; visualizing yourself performing the task confidently and competently

♦**Kinesthetic:** the movements associated with a task: feeling the contact with your equipment, opposing players, the field, the pool, and the ice

♦**Gustatory:** tastes connected with an activity: the water, sweat

♦**Olfactory:** smells linked with performance: chalk, grass, leather, chlorine, etc.

♦**Auditory:** the sounds associated with performance: hearing the sound of the ball making contact with your racquet, the splash of the water as you dive into the pool, your skate blade on the ice, the bat hitting your ball, etc.

You are engaged in a training run down a street close to your home on a crisp autumn day. You feel the cold bite of the air in your nose and throat as you breathe in large gulps of air. You are running easily and smoothly; but you feel pleasantly tired and can feel your heart pounding in your chest. Your leg muscles are tired, especially the calf and thigh; and you can feel your feet slapping against the pavement. As you run, you can feel a warm sweat on your body.

This description of the runner's physical and emotional responses to the run provides a useful model for response-laden compositions. Encourage students to create imagery scripts that sensationalize an experience or performance. Imagine yourself diving into the water. Picture yourself getting ready to perform the action. Recreate the physical and emotional tension associated with standing on the edge of the pool. Capture the thrill and exuberance of a skillful and graceful dive, as you become aware of the sensations around you (the sounds of other people in the pool, the water lapping onto the deck, the smell of the chlorine). Feel how your whole body is engaged in the experience— your heart, your muscles, your lungs, your inner being. Live in the

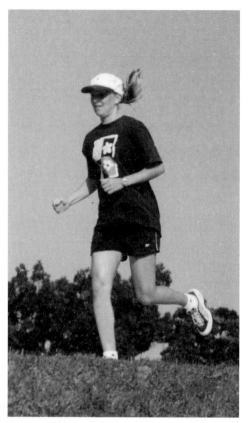

Think about what you feel.

middle of the action; become absorbed by it. Revel in the joy of streaming through the water, a million bubbles jetting along beside you as you glide into the depths of the pool and then back to the surface. According to Lang, Kozak, Miller, Lavin, and McLean (1980), instruction based on response-laden compositions produces stronger physiological responses than does instruction that depends on stimulus-laden imagery. However, combining stimulus- and response-laden compositions offers learners rich imagery scripts, and the best results in performance.

How Does Imagery Work?

Imagery promotes elaboration. It allows the learner to preview and review performance and the conditions and emotions that surround performance. Through imagery, learners can visit and revisit situations, recreate the emotional build-up and challenge, and then mentally script how their performance will unfold. Imagery may also help alter or subdue details about the environment. For example, if spectators hinder performance, the performer can imagine turning down the noise of the spectators as if lowering the volume on a radio, or blur the focus on their faces the way a photographer might blur the background to enhance the distinctiveness of the primary subject.

Moritz, Hall, Martin, and Vadocz (1996) suggest that imaged rehearsal of specific skills may not be as important as imagery of sports-related experiences and emotions in building athletic confidence. Participants should reproduce in their minds not only a masterful performance but also the range of experiences that surround it and the confident emotions that precede, accompany, and follow upon it. Developing an appropriate script for imagery requires an elaborate staging of the task. It is therefore important to rehearse the conditions that instigate a performance, the emotions that surround the event, as well as the performance itself. The teacher cannot create this script for learners. Using examples of such imagery scripts, however, will enable learners to craft

Types of Imagery

Internal	External
Performers see, feel, hear, and taste the experience through his/her own eyes. When you experience an action internally, you see the action as if with an internal video camera. You see, for example, the ball travelling towards you as a performer.	When you stand back mentally from yourself in performing a skill you witness your performance externally. It is as if you are a spectator sitting in the stands watching yourself.

their own scripts.

Imagery in Sport

My work as a gymnastics coach has convinced me that imagery can be a powerful tool. Before I ever read much of the technical literature on imagery, I was encouraging my gymnasts (ages 10-14) to "see" the movements and to "feel" themselves explode off the floor or the vault. I used to tell them to imagine that a series of strobe photographs were out in front of them and that as they ran forward they should try to imagine they were collecting the images along with their power and grace. When they hit the end of the runway they were to explode with the force and concentration of all the images they had collected. Some of the gymnasts related unusual experiences on different occasions. When one gymnast who had completed a particularly difficult 'trick' on the floor with amazing height and precision, she asked: "Did I do it?" Apparently, she had concentrated so intensely on the image in her head that she was unaware of what was happening to her, or that she had executed her element with such success. She had experienced what Csikszentmihalyi (1990) refers to as an "optimal experience ...when a person's body or mind is stretched to its limits in a voluntary effort to accomplish something difficult and worthwhile."

It is worth noting here that optimal experience is something we can make happen: with the right tools, we can improve performance

Benefits of using Imagery:

♦increase concentration

♦enhance focus on the key elements of performance

♦block out distractions

♦enliven learning

♦involve students in the learning process

dramatically. Not every performance is spectacular or reaches great heights. However, with practice, all learners can be more deliberate and methodical about the way they approach learning a skill. The integration of imagery into a regular physical education program has great promise and has implications for the way classes are structured and managed.

Imagery in Physical Education

Effective teachers find ways of actively engaging students in the learning process. This not only encourages them to dedicate their time, both in and out of school, to practice, but also teaches them to be responsible and self-reliant. Imagery enhances control because it enables learners to:

Create a stable image of the performance During the early stages of learning, performance may be erratic and inconsistent. A stable image or mental blueprint of the performance enables learners to compare performance to selected standards and make on-going adjustments.

Selectively filter information Especially during the early stages of learning, students may feel overwhelmed by information and stimulus. Imagery can help learners concentrate on key aspects of performance.

Develop a conceptual plan of action Imagining movement sequences prior to an actual performance helps to anticipate, rehearse, and review achievement.

Cope with challenges Performers can act out specific situations and strategies in their heads. Orlick (1986) refers to this process as testing the circuits. Seeing oneself executing a strategy, in the context of 'real' play, is an important way of bridging practice and game play. Visualizing oneself confidently, accurately reading and reacting to one's opponents, and coping with distractions such as crowd noise are also important when preparing for an activity.

Keep sharp during layoff periods Mental performance of a skill can help students keep psychologically and kinesthetically sharp during lay-offs and injury or idle periods. Imagery enhances retention in the absence of actual performance. It can be practiced without equipment, at any time, in any place, and does not fatigue the person.

Improves the speed and quality of skill development Imagery does two important things for teachers. First, it encourages learners to think (plan, rehearse, reflect) about a movement before and after it is executed. Second, it gives students more control over practice. By providing themselves with cues, analysis, and feedback, imagery users take an active responsibility in improving their performance.

Change beliefs and attitudes The use of imagery requires students who consider themselves poor performers to cast themselves in roles that are highly successful. Self-doubt, nervousness, fear, and impulsivity hinder performance. Imagery provides you an opportunity to overcome these obstacles and to convince yourself that you can indeed execute the task successfully.

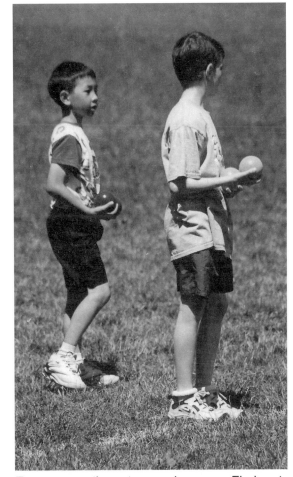

Encourage others to use imagery. Find out what images work for others.

Induce relaxation Imagery works best when the body and the mind are relaxed. The ability to relax is an important skill. Relaxation before performance reduces energy loss, blocks out distractions, builds confidence, and focuses attention on the essential components of performance that result in success (Suinn, 1980).

Imagery works best when the representations are:

Performed in a relaxed state Ensure that the learner is mentally and physically relaxed before using imagery to strengthen performance. Teach imagery protocols that include a period of time prior to performance devoted to relaxing the body and the mind in preparation for imagery rehearsal.

Meaningful Images that are vivid, specific, and relevant to the learner are more likely to have a positive impact on the learner. What is vivid to one student may be ambiguous to another. It is therefore important that teachers work with students to create explicit mental images of the performance. Continue to probe for responses that will indicate what and how a learner sees, feels, and hears the movement or activity.

Performed in their entirety Imagine the task or activity from beginning to end. This entails a thorough awareness of all facts of the experience, e.g., the movement or skill itself, coping with unexpected situations, giving 100%, the emotional arousal of the challenge, the feelings of confidence, the response by onlookers, the response of the teacher, etc.

Performed in real time Although students may derive some benefit from slow motion imagery to analyze a skill, it is better to imagine its execution in real time in order to replicate the speed and timing-related features of the experience.

Positive Imagine a performance that is successful and competent. Too often, learners bombard themselves with negative images. Avoid this mistake: imagine a successful performance.

Practiced in conjunction with physical performance Imagery alone is not as effective as imagery combined with physical practice. Follow an imagery session with a physical performance of the skill.

Imagery is like having a replay camera in your head, except YOU get to create what happens!

Experienced using as many senses as possible during the imagery episode Make the experience 'alive' visually, kinesthetically, and auditorily.

Fun Keep the imagery experience interesting and enjoyable. Use terms and situations learners find appealing. Encourage them to apply the techniques to areas beyond skill performance.

Integrated into the teaching/learning process Although it may be taught initially as a separate skill, imagery should be incorporated into skill development as soon as possible. Students will better appreciate the connection between strategy use and skill learning.

Understood relative to the learner Students need to define imagery and its benefits in their own terms. They should be encouraged to describe the procedures that work best for them, and the ways in which imagery benefits their own learning and relates to different learning situations.

Modeled by teachers and other learners Models not only convey procedures but also help win acceptance. Moreover, peer models communicate a sense of confidence and healthy competition: "If she can do it, so can I!"

Previously experienced Sensory awareness of the task facilitates imagery. The better skill you command, the more able you are to use imagery related to the skill. In other words, as a skill improves so also does the imagery.

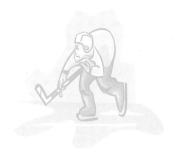

Focused on performance mastery Picture yourself excelling in performance. Imagine yourself as the most technically proficient performer.

Taught progressively in combination with other skills Imagery

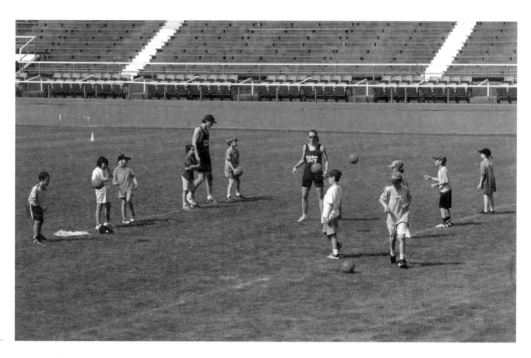

Blend strategy use into instruction and practice.

skills should be developed through increasingly complex routines in conjunction with other skills, such as throwing, shooting, etc.

Incorporated into daily living Learning at school should not be isolated from life outside school. Encourage students to use imagery to manage daily living during play, in academic pursuits, at home, to resolve conflicts, when experiencing fear, coping with stress, etc.

Learning to Use Imagery

Since imagery is first learned as a separate skill, instruction about its use should begin in a classroom setting. Here students have a chance to experience imagery as a unique form of awareness. They can then explore different types of imagery and relate them to daily activities. Imagery exercises can be used to develop both skill and confidence in creating imagery scripts and sequences. It should be applied to learning or refining a skill as soon as possible.

As new features of the use of imagery are mastered they should be integrated into the entire learning process. In an imagery learning program students begin by developing an understanding of how and why it is important to create vivid images (comprehension). Next, they practice forming vivid images in a variety of everyday situations – imagining a story before it is written (consolidation). Immediately following, they learn to create vivid images in relation to specific movement patterns – the overhand throw (application). Finally, students are encouraged to help others adopt the techniques they have mastered (consultation). Workshop sheets for such a program are included in the appendix. They are designed to introduce students to the study and use of imagery to improve their thinking skills and their skill acquisition. Each phase of the program is designed to deepen understanding of imagery as a tool for learning and to demonstrate how teachers can advance the study of imagery and its use in physical education.

Phase 1: Comprehension

Students need experience and time to understand how to exercise some measure of control over the details and events that are occurring in their minds and bodies. Prior to actually talking and thinking about imagery, the first few lessons should focus on movement stories.

Sample Activity for the Classroom #1

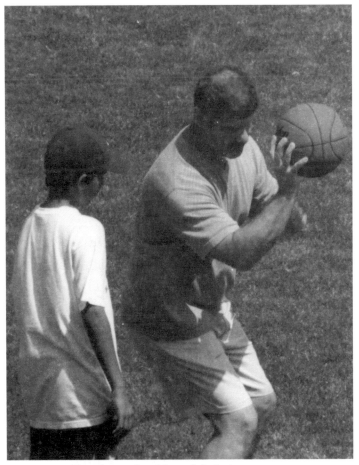

Teachers should model strategy use.

On flash cards, display action words such as pop, dash, flop, skip, hop, or slide. Ask the students to think about the movements they will perform to represent the words. Instruct the students to: "see the action in your mind." Then, after pausing for a moment have them show it. After several trials, students can be instructed to make up a movement story for a partner who will try to name the

Phases of Learning

Comprehension: What is imagery? Why should I be interested in imagery? What is the most effective way to image?

Consolidation: How can I use imagery consistently, effectively, and routinely?

Application: How should I apply the use of imagery to learning new skills?

Consultation: How do I reflect on my own progress and share ideas about imagery and skill development with others?

movements describing the actions. Students can then prepare flash cards of their own.

Sample Activity for the Classroom #2

Present a movement story about a person making a snowman, who then becomes the snowman, and proceeds to melt under the hot sun. Students are instructed to think of a movement story, plan the body actions that will depict the story, and then perform it for their partners. Young students are quite adept and willing to be involved in the creation and performance of elaborate and dramatic movement stories. Extension into the language arts program should be quite natural. Conversely, stories prepared in language arts classes can be used in physical education classes to enrich both programs. Other movement stories might show: barbecuing, washing the car, painting, fishing, downhill skiing, etc.

We started our hike up a steep hill. The back pack we were carrying was extremely heavy so we had to lean into the hill... .

Sample Activity for the Classroom #3

Students need to explore how to develop clear, vivid images and how to control them. Exercises should be enjoyable and practical. For example, students can become familiar with imagery that is highly visual and tactile by imagining that they are lying on a bed of marshmallows. Not a complex activity, this use of imagery nevertheless should enable students to discover the ways in which ideas flow from the experience, as well as the power of the mind. Students will then be eager to try other exercises.

Phase 2: Consolidation

Students need plenty of time and a variety of occasions for using imagery to refine their understanding of its scope and character and to recognize its diversity and importance. Students can experiment with imagery techniques (e.g., making imagined objects larger, smaller, viewed from above or below, etc.). Most students enjoy manipulating objects, ideas, and emotions in their heads. These exercises can be included as part of daily activities before and during physical education classes, writing and drama classes, visual art, as well as music classes. Imagery should be seen as an important way of preparing students for activities that involve concentration, creativity, and the coordination of thought and action. In combination with relaxation exercises, imagery consolidation activities provide an opportunity to explore the underlying layers of imagery in many different situations.

Phase 3: Application

This phase involves directing learners to use imagery for specific purposes. In physical education, imagery is used as a tool to help learners focus on specific body actions, control objects, avoid distractions, and centre on specific goals. Students should be encouraged to develop a ritual or routine for imagery. For example, just before going up to bat in baseball, close your eyes and visualize the proper stance, swing, and follow through. As you imagine the action, it is best to stand back from your physical surroundings both physically and mentally. Retreat to 'another world' for a moment as you mentally prepare for performance. The teacher needs to model these actions frequently. Examples from the sports world can also show students that athletes of all ages prepare for peak performances by using imagery. Invite local sports personalities to share the conversations, stories, and images that help them perform optimally.

Phase 4: Consultation

Students who are able to describe and explain the use of imagery to their friends have reached the final stage. Their accounts of using imagery to control performance and emotion are so well understood by this point, they are able to coach others. In some instances, students are able to convince classmates of the merits of imagery and provide suggestions for ways of improving performance using imagery. But working with peers should be extended to the comprehension, consolidation, and application phases as well, thereby facilitating this last phase of consultation. For example, during the comprehension phase, instruct students to tell their partners what they imagined when they tried making their room at home change colours. Encourage students to participate in class discussion and to write down their stories. Recognizing the highly personal character of the imagery process gives students the impetus to be creative and open about their own learning habits, preferences, strengths, and weaknesses.

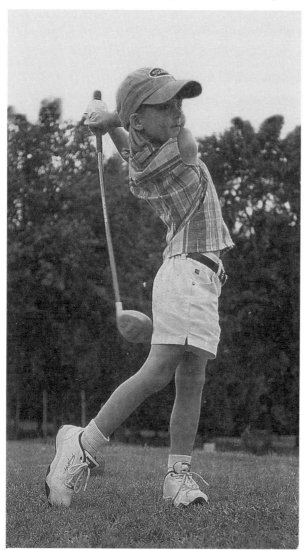

Strategy use is good for everyone. Think, do, review.

Program Goals and Expectations

The learning workshop activity sheets (see appendix) are designed to be used by teachers to help students advance through the various phases of imagery use towards self-regulated learning. These sheets can also be distributed to students for use as another part of a home study program. For example, the teacher may introduce the idea of using your imagination to see body actions and to control body movements. Students could then use the sheets to work on the techniques themselves to heighten awareness and to facilitate their routine application. During each class, the teacher can set time aside for discussing the use of imagery and its application to

Good Imagery Users:

- **Incorporate** as many senses as possible to represent the action

- **Focus** on quality first

- **See** themselves as the doer in the images

- **Focus** on their responses, not the outcomes

- **Are** able to manipulate and control the images, and thus change their performance as needed

- **Practice** imagery every day

- **Extend** imagery to relaxation as well as the performance of skills

- **Apply** imagery techniques to daily living

- **See** the action in real time

- **Keep** track of how they image, so that in personalizing the use of imagery, they come to know how imagery works for them

skill improvement and for sharing student insights. Like any new skill, the use of imagery takes time and practice to master. But introduced early in elementary school and maintained through the secondary school years, imagery use can become an integral part of the learning process. The following verbal sequence should become a routine part of both instruction and practice: Imagine it! Try it! Think about it! Try again!

Handouts and Workshop Activities for Students

A unit organized around the use of imagery in a physical education class might include the following:

Rationale Imagery use enables learners to assume more control over the thought processes associated with learning new physical skills and using them. Imagery users are more focused and deliberate about their performances. Experienced in physical education classes, imagery can be applied to learning and achievement in other settings: visual arts, music, creative writing, drama, mathematics, communication, and

Imagine it!
Try it!
Think back about it!
Try again!

Characteristics of Good Imagery Users

Vividness

Good imagery users sensationalize their portrayal of an experience. They can:

♦ **see it:** are able to imagine body parts, body part movement, imagine from an internal perspective, put the motions in context, depict movements in relation to positive outcomes, and view their experiences in colour

♦ **feel it:** are able physically and emotionally to experience the body action and their responses to the environments around them (coldness), and to sense the texture of the things they come in contact with

♦ **hear it:** are able to create the various sounds of the experience in the environment: cheering crowds, themselves engaged in the activity (water splashing over their body), and the people around them (running footsteps)

♦ **smell it:** are aware of the smell of the surroundings related to the experience (chlorine in a pool) and the equipment

♦ **taste it:** are able to taste, for example, the snow and spray of ice, the sweat from their brow, and the water consumed during the event

Control

Good imagery users can manipulate and control their images, viewing the experience from different:

♦ **perspectives:** internal, external

♦ **ratios:** smaller, larger, narrow, wide, long, short

♦ **vantage points:** as a tiny insect, from the ceiling, peeking out from a closet, from above and below

♦ **directions:** forward, backward, sideways

♦ **rotations:** right, left, front to back, back to front

♦ **replications:** divide in half, double

♦ **weights:** heavy, light

♦ **temperatures:** cold, hot

♦ **speeds:** slow, fast, actual

♦ **emotions:** happy, confident

♦ **fluidity:** smooth, fragmented

creative thinking activities. The use of imagery can be used to help manage stress, cope with stress, and plan for success. Imagery use is a life skill.

Outcome   Students use imagery to enhance skill development.

It is expected that the learners will:

1. Use all five senses to image, with clarity and control:
- ◆body positions (standing, sitting, floating)
- ◆body actions (walking, running, rolling)
- ◆object control (catching, throwing, kicking)
- ◆object manipulation (rotating, enlarging, miniaturizing)
- ◆feelings (happiness/sadness, anxiety/relaxation, confidence/ fear, heaviness/lightness, roughness/smoothness, cold/heat, pain/comfort, tightness/looseness, wetness/dryness, slipperiness/abrasiveness, wood, plants, steel, plastic, leather, cloth, etc.)
- ◆sounds (breathing, running pattern, dog barking)
- ◆smells (leaves in autumn, water in a swimming pool, leather baseball glove, cooking)
- ◆taste (snow, salt water, favourite foods)

2. Explain imagery in their own words to:
- ◆ define its character and scope
- ◆ describe how it promotes achievement

3. Use imagery to enhance skill development of :
- ◆ fundamental movement patterns (throwing, kicking, catching)
- ◆ specialized movement patterns (running a pattern and catching a ball)

4. Use imagery to self-regulate movement by:
- ◆ planning movement
- ◆ monitoring movement in relation to intended outcomes
- ◆ assessing performance
- ◆ analyzing movement
- ◆ solving movement problems

5. Apply imagery skills to daily life in order to:

   ♦ regulate emotions
   ♦ cope with stress
   ♦ learn new skills

Imagery Summary

Imagery is a powerful way to rehearse body actions in your mind. It gives the learner a chance to practice the movements, replay performance, and to analyze execution. It can also be a way to motivate involvement, reduce anxiety, and prepare for participation. Imagery is a way to carefully script intention and anticipate engagement. Imagery should be practiced regularly and with the same care devoted to physical practice.

"Follow through like that."

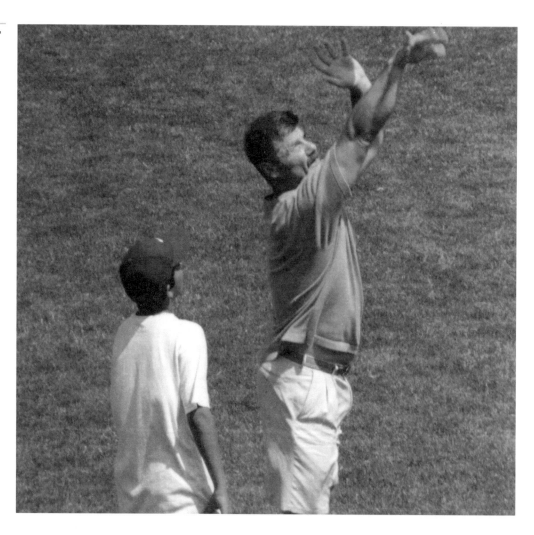

Building Understanding

♦ What does the effectiveness of imagery suggest about the learning process?

♦ What can teachers learn about the involvement of learners in the learning process through the use of imagery?

♦ What is the role of the teacher and the student in the use of imagery?

♦ What are different ways imagery can be used to enhance learning?

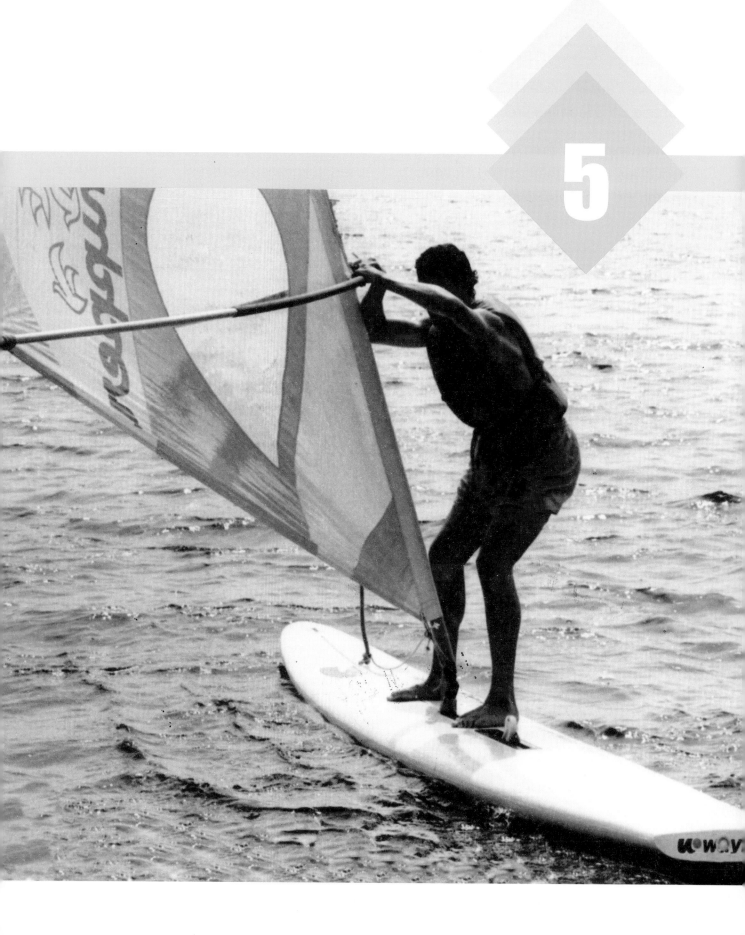

5

SELF-TALK

Chapter Objectives

Define self-talk

◇

Distinguish different kinds of self-talk

◇

Describe the benefits of self-talk

◇

Relate self-talk use to learning

◇

Relate self-talk use to self-reliant learning

◇

Teach self-talk use

◇

Use classroom ready materials to build skills for self-talk and self-reliant learning

Self-talk is our 'inner voice.' It is important to interact with our own thoughts.

◇

Definition of Self-talk

The next time you parallel park, follow a recipe, look for a book in the library, or talk yourself into or out of a trip to the dessert table, listen to the conversations you are having with yourself. People frequently and instinctively use self-talk as an internal guidance system. Everyday self-talk can help control emotions, promote logical and reasoned thinking, regulate task performance, or help us cope with challenging situations.

Self-talk involves the use of words, phrases, or sentences spoken aloud or privately in order to direct preparation, execution, analysis, and feedback while learning a skill. The term self-talk has been used in different ways by various researchers. For example, Vygotsky (1962) uses the term "private speech" to refer to the dialogue we have with ourselves in consciously directing, monitoring, and reflecting on our behaviour. Verbal rehearsal and self-instruction are other terms used to describe self-talk when it is used to plan thoughts or guide behaviour (Meichenbaum, 1977; Weiss, 1983).

Unlike cues and labels, self-talk is the process of consciously and deliberately interacting orally with oneself in order to direct a specific action or behaviour. Cues and labels tend to be teacher-directed prompts. Whether and how the learner interacts with these prompts depends on how the students handle the messages cognitively. An example of teacher-directed labelling or cueing is the use of the acronym 'BEEF' to help students focus on the key elements of shooting a basketball: Balance, Elbow, Elevation, Follow-through. Self-talk, however, is scripted communication between the learner and him/herself, in a dialogue perhaps such as the following: "OK, before I shoot I need to get balanced, feet shoulder-width apart; ya, that feels solid." The learner thus incorporates what has been presented in class (e.g., what it means to take a balanced position). Self-talk can also contain picture words and imagery. In fact, it is difficult not to blend the two together. Back to the basketball shot: "OK, get balanced – if I were standing on a teeter-tottcr would I tip? Good, that feels solid. Now, take a moment and let me review the actions I want my body to perform ..." I tell my students self-talk is like having your own special teacher working alongside you.

What is so special about the teacher is that it's YOU.

Benefits of Self-talk

Self talk can be the teacher's window into the cognitive processes at work inside a learner's head. Self-talk can help teachers determine specific difficulties a learner may be experiencing. For example, most beginners caution themselves when they ski not to hit trees, people, or other objects. Seldom do they script verbally what is required for an accident-free run. Physical education teachers rely heavily on language and demonstration to communicate information. In turn, they expect students to use language and demonstration to express their understanding of the material presented. A limited vocabulary may force less skilled learners to be passive because they don't have the vocabulary and the technical expertise to express themselves. Self-talk, along with picture words, enables students to develop a language of picture words that fosters a more insightful and detailed exchange of ideas between learners and the teacher.

Benefits of Self-talk:

- boosts confidence
- aids recall
- narrows focus of attention
- resists negative thinking
- cues performance

  Self-talk can help learners plan and monitor their cognitive activity, which in turn can regulate and enhance motor performance. Learners construct movement plans (first I take a step, then I turn my hips), then they try them out and compare what they performed with what they expected to achieve. Every learner's results will be somewhat different from the model presented - it is only natural. No two bodies are exactly alike; no two brains work in the same way. Therefore, it is up to the learner to work along with the teacher through the process. This is why strategy use is so exciting. Students and teachers learn to explore the way sense is constructed together. Students should be encouraged to question how skills are developed, how their bodies work, and how they can customize to make the skill work for them. Increased awareness of the learning process preserves self esteem by explicitly teaching children to recognize the factors responsible for failure, such as inattentiveness, fatigue, lack of knowledge of task requirements, and so on.

  Self-talk also promotes a deliberate and systematic approach to learning. Because learners have a clear sense of purpose, they are able to function more independently, competently, and confidently. Perhaps the most important result of using any strategy is that the users come to regard themselves as capable learners. When this occurs, persistence and effort increase and the likelihood of achievement is usually not far behind.

Kinds of Self-talk

We use self-talk in all kinds of situations. Two stories provide examples of how self-talk can be used to cope with anxiety, focus on alternative and positive images, and control our emotions.

Too often, everyday conversations with ourselves are negative or full of self-doubt or chastisement. Often, I hear people say to themselves, "Don't be so stupid," or "That wasn't a very bright move, was it?" or "You'll never get this done on time." With a little practice, negative self-talk can be converted into a productive and praise-oriented pep talk: "I can overcome this. I know that if I focus on watching the ball make contact with the racquet, I'll hit it better.") .

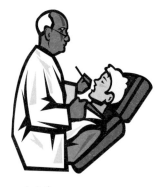

Sports-related Self-talk

Self-talk in a sport setting can be a powerful tool. Unfortunately, most people do not consciously construct a self-talk conversation or script that could prompt and guide their performance. Instead, positive self-talk is replaced by an irate coach, a nagging doubter on the sidelines, or

Kathy's Story

A friend recently told me how she uses self-talk when visiting the dentist. Dental visits make her nervous. To prepare for the visit she tells herself the dentist is her friend, that she has conquered much bigger challenges, and that to be afraid of going to the dentist is 'childish.' During the visit she works on controlling her breathing and visually imaging quiet, restful scenes from trips she has enjoyed. Her use of self-talk and imagery allows her to complete the visit without conveying to the dentist and the other patients that she is terrified. She has developed a specific routine or plan for dental visits that involves conversations with self and mental imagery for relaxation.

Denise's Story

While touring the exhibits, her daughter noticed that one of the zoo personnel was carrying a large snake to a display area. Quickly, a crowd gathered and her daughter wanted to join the crowd. But the mother hated snakes; her heart began to race, her face flushed, and although she realized she was in a difficult situation, she did not want to convey this fear to her daughter lest she develop the same phobia. She began to converse with herself, "What should I do, Melissa wants to see the snake. My God what if I faint or panic? OK, get yourself under control. What would a calm, interested parent say in this situation? This snake is not venomous and the keeper is in control. OK, let her approach the snake, not me." She turned to her daughter and in a voice she thought was firm and confident said: "Go ahead Melissa, stand over there by the other girls and I will stay back here to leave room for other children to see." She did not attempt to deny her extreme fear of snakes; instead, she decided to focus on controlling her emotional responses. Her approach was successful, she got to stay away from the snake, gave her daughter a chance to learn more about snakes, and avoided having her daughter witness her mother become too fearful or disturbed.

In this case self-talk helped:
- organize her thoughts
- focus on preferred behaviour and speech patterns

a disappointed partner.

In addition to helping them understand that they are in charge of the situation, self-talk encourages people to be more performance-oriented. Said differently, the golfer below (see box on next page) needed to pay closer attention to what he was supposed to do to swing the club well, rather than focusing on missing the water or hitting the green. Used properly, self-talk prompts the performer to be more analytical, planned, and methodical in relation to the means rather than the outcomes or ends of an action. Using self-talk, performers realize that outcomes are a function of their ability to control their own actions. Rather than blaming the design of the golf course, the clubs, the ball, the wind, or any other excuse, Brian can concentrate on what he needs to do to swing well, regardless of the situation.

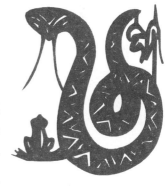

Another example can help illustrate the same concept. An agile

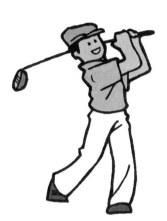

eight-year-old gymnast was having difficulty doing cartwheels on the balance beam. Fine on the low beam, she consistently fell off when she moved up to the regulation height. When asked what was on her mind as she tried to perform the cartwheel, she replied, "I think about not hurting myself when I fall off." We went back to the low beam and I asked her to tell me what advice she would give a fellow gymnast about cartwheels on the beam. She immediately said, "Don't worry, it's just like a cartwheel on the floor except you have to grasp the beam tightly." We talked about the important features of the cartwheel - the straight and tight body, the arms pushing the body tall and directing the flow, and the first foot reaching for the beam. Together we put together a movement script for the cartwheel: "Tight and tall, reach for the beam, squeeze it, stretch tall, place the foot, and push." I stood beside the high beam as she coached herself through a couple of cartwheels, providing a light spot each time. Eventually, she became so absorbed in repeating and following her own instructions that she didn't notice that I was no

Brian's Story

On the golf course, I listen to what my friends say to themselves in certain situations. The seventh hole on this particular golf course is 125 yards to the green. Just before the green is a water pond that stretches across the entire fairway. Evergreen trees skirt the back of the green and sand bunkers are on either side of the trees. As my friend Brian approached the tee, I overheard this conversation: "This is the nastiest hole on the course. They do this just to ruin a perfectly good round. Well, let's see if I can find an old ball. No sense loosing a good one in the drink." If I were to ask Brian for a lesson on how to hit the ball with a nine iron, he would be able to give me an extensive description. He has seen several hundred nine iron shots live and on television, so his mental image of a good nine iron shot is probably well established. However, he has not been able to get his golf swing together with his thinking. What if he changed his self-talk to: "Great, this is the hole that teaches me about concentration and good form under pressure. OK, what am I supposed to remember to do to swing well? My stance is good, head down, focus on the dimples, soft body, easy back, and smooth through the ball." Even if he is unsuccessful, at least he knows what he did, rather than what the course did to him. He needs to understand that he is in control.

longer spotting her. Occasionally, she still falls; but now she realizes that it is because she is not focusing properly, not because she can't perform the cartwheel. If students in any sport or activity can learn how to manage the thought processes involved in controlling their body movements, they will be able to monitor their own performances, compare their actions against the standards they have set for themselves, make the necessary changes, persist in their efforts—and attribute gains to their own efforts and abilities.

Self-talk for Learning

Self-talk should become an integral part of the learning process. It can heighten awareness of the key elements of form that characterize mature, successful performance. Self-talk may also serve to highlight a learner's preferences. For example, some self-talkers prefer to use words that conjure up particular images, while others prefer words that are connected to particular sounds or feelings. When I teach young children how to catch, I give them a choice of words that will remind them to flex their arms as the catch is made. Some children like the words "soft," "cushion," or "pillow," while others get better results when they say "Make the catch as quiet as possible." Still others like the idea of the arms "vacuuming" the ball into their body with their arms. Each word conjures up images and sensations the children can relate to personally and use effectively to guide their practice. I remember two young students who created an elaborate drama to help them learn the catching action. They created a scenario with bean bags representing airplanes approaching an aircraft carrier. They made sound effects to go with the approach, the opening of the carrier platform, and the landing. As the planes landed they vacuumed the planes onto the deck of their imaginary carriers. They were totally absorbed by the story and worked diligently, needing virtually no additional instruction. I asked them to tell me their story to see if they had created a situation that would prompt the proper action. Satisfied that conceptually they had the 'right' idea, I watched them practice. Both were 'zoned' in on the flight of the ball. I praised them for creating such an

Good Self-talkers:

♦ accept that self-talk is a normal and powerful way to enhance learning and performance

♦ include picture words in their self-talk monologues

♦ use positive self-talk

♦ keep the conversations short

♦ focus on quality

♦ plan what to say to be effective

♦ evaluate what they say and do

♦ apply self-talk to daily living

effective story, for remembering the key elements of form, and for working so skillfully and thoughtfully on the task. Later, they shared their story with the rest of the class.

The language that is used in the self-talk conversations enables students to communicate effectively with each other and their teacher. Metaphors and analogies (picture words) can be substituted for technical terms. Movement stories are an even more elaborate version of picture words. Picture words enable learners and teachers to talk about skills using everyday experiences and terms. Students ask better questions: "Watch my wings of the eagle. Am I holding them right?" versus "What am I doing wrong?" In the first instance, the learner has already engaged in a process of mentally matching form with the demonstration and explanation provided previously and now held in the mind's eye. This is an important step towards achieving greater independence. The second question ("What am I doing wrong?") suggests the learner expects the teacher to conduct the analysis and to correct what needs fixing, thereby remaining dependent on the teacher.

At the end of a lesson I often demonstrate the skill with distinct common errors. I then ask the students to give me some advice about how to improve the skill. They are quite adept at identifying, demonstrating, and correcting my performance. They are excited by their new found sense of power over the skill and their capacity to serve as an instructor to themselves, to others—not to mention their teacher.

Instructional self-talk is an attempt to use self-talk to channel thinking towards improving the quality of the skill. Initially, learners may struggle to find the right words to describe key elements of a particular movement. This is understandable, since most people are not equipped to study movement as precisely as the experts. The teacher can overcome knowledge gaps by preparing a sample 'movement story' or script to describe complex body actions (induced self-talk) or students can create their own scripts once they learn the key elements of form (personalized self-talk). Instructional self-talk must be purposeful and process-oriented. Instructional self-talk focuses on questions that enable learners to think more carefully about their actions.

What is the learner trying to do?

What is the action sequence: what do I do first, second . . .,
and what do I do last?

How am I thinking about this: do I have the right picture
words and images in my mind?

What should I try to remember next time?

Induced self-talk is self-talk using the words, phrases and ideas created or scripted by someone else. Induced self-talk may be necessary for several reasons. First, learners may not think to use the self-talk technique on their own. Second, they may not know enough about the skill to select the appropriate metaphors and analogies to use in their self-talk script. Third, they may be so overwhelmed by the onslaught of information and challenge before them that they cannot gather their thoughts into an organized plan for success. Fourth, although all of us have used self-talk at some time, many among us may not have used self-talk properly or strategically.

Personalized self-talk Words, phrases, and conversations are the scripted terms, internal dialogues, and/or movement stories fashioned by learners to describe a body action. After students become comfortable using self-talk and are convinced of its merit, they will begin to invent their own terms. No matter how carefully we try to repeat a story told to us by someone else, we invariably elaborate, embellish or personalize the information. Why? Because new ideas are interpreted relative to our previous experiences. We remember the meaning or gist of the story by putting events into a context to which we can relate. Rather than denying that learners are constructing their own versions of the information presented in class, teachers should look for ways of encouraging and sharing these insights. Invite children to give their version of what they see. For example, to prepare for the 'throw in' for soccer, the ball is held between both hands forming a 'W' with the thumbs. Stand with the feet shoulder width apart and the arms extended overhead. This extended body is arched backwards and then vigorously thrust forward as the ball is released. Initially, I asked the students to tell themselves to "stretch tall, arch, and then explode forward." Later, I asked the children to tell me what they thought would help them remember what to do at each phase of the throw-in. One student suggested naming the first part of the skill "i" because the body is straight and tall and the dot over the 'i' represented the ball. Another child suggested the arch be represented by a "backwards 'C'" and the follow through by a "right way 'C'." A large piece of chart paper had already been put up on the wall to record the children's ideas about other skills. As learners, they were developing a vocabulary and language that would allow them to exchange ideas and confirm whether the action presented matched the images discussed. More importantly, it gave the learners permission to define movement using their own terms.

If personalized self-talk does not occur naturally, prompt students to create picture words and movement stories to describe body actions. After demonstrating a particular movement, ask the students for picture words that would describe the action. The teacher must carefully direct students to the key features of the performance requiring description.

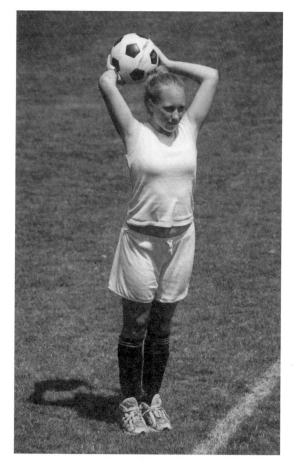

For example, if you want the students to give you picture words to describe the elongated step action prior to stepping beside the soccer ball, have them attend specifically to this action.

Self-talk in Physical Education

Self-talk, imagery, and picture words work hand-in-hand in the learning process in physical education. In order to select, arrange, and verbalize the phrases, stories, and words learners must use in self-talk, attention must be focused on the language and action. This conjunction amplifies and intensifies the cognitive and metacognitive activity necessary for learning improvement. When I'm telling myself to get ready to do a forward roll, "hands on the floor like spider webs, roll on my shoulder, look at my belly button (look for lint), heels on my bum," I don't have much room in my head for any distract-

How You Do It

Teacher:	"Watch what I do with my legs as I approach the ball."
	"What does that look like to you?"
	"Have you ever seen that action before?"
	"Mary, what did you see?"
Mary:	"Well, to me it looked like a leap."
Teacher:	"Any other ideas?" "Jeff?"
Jeff:	"To me, it looked like a pair of scissors opening."
Teacher:	"Watch the leg action again a couple of times and see if Mary's and Jeff's pictures fit."
Teacher:	"Return to the space where you were working before and teach yourself using self-talk. I will come around and ask you which words best helped you remember what to do."

ing thoughts. This enables me to be more concentrated and determined about what I am doing. Indeed, I can coach myself; I know what I am supposed to do. If you recall the opening paragraph to this chapter, I made reference to parallel parking. A person who talks to him/herself, has taken charge of the situation allowing him/her to direct both thought and action towards a specific task. Self-talk is like

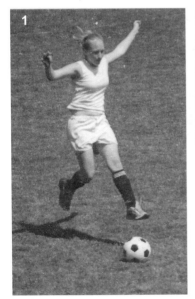

"Jump to it."

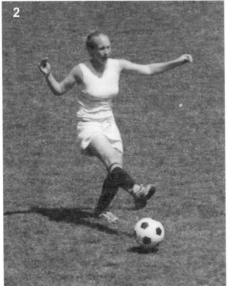

Use self-talk to cue the action, "Use big foot."

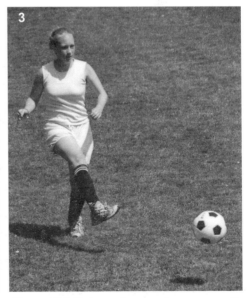

Use self-talk to review performance—"I need to remember to step into the ball."

Self-talk is like turning up the volume on the radio so all other information is blocked out and only the transmitter's message is heard.

turning up the volume on the radio so all other information is blocked out and only the transmitter's message is heard.

Other Applications of Self-talk

Instructional self-talk has been used effectively in both clinical and instructional settings for nearly two decades. Self-talk has helped subjects control aggressive and impulsive behavior and cope with phobias (Meichenbaum, 1977), facilitate problem-solving in mathematics (Schonfeld, 1983), improve writing skills (Englert, Raphael, Anderson, Anthony, & Stevens, 1991), and manage performance stress among elite athletes (Orlick, 1986). Recent theoretical accounts of learning, which view learners as active seekers and thinkers, have considered the use of self-talk as a means of monitoring how individuals perceive and process information (Brown & Palinscar, 1989), a way of training subjects in the development and use of metacognitive skills (Chi & Bassock, 1989; Brown & Palinscar, 1989), and a means of enhancing self-confidence in relation to skill performance (Schunk, 1991).

Self-talk and Self-regulated Learning

Schunk (1986) reviewed the relationship between verbalization (self-talk) and children's learning and concluded that verbalization helps children (especially those who have difficulty attending to or recalling information) self-regulate cognitive skills such as attending, coding, associating, rehearsing, and monitoring. Additionally, self-talk enhances the learner's capacity to code, store, and retain information that the learner can recall for use in applied situations. It also helps students focus their attention on the important features of a task, rather than irrelevant information (Schunk, 1991; Landin, 1994).

According to Fuson (1979) verbal rehearsal serves to focus selectively children's attention on task-appropriate cues and helps them remember what to do. Fuson affirmed that for children seven years of age and younger who do not spontaneously rehearse information, prompting them to rehearse verbally appears to be a necessary procedure for effective motor reproduction. Weiss and Klint (1987) found similar results in a gymnasium setting. Self-talk used as a systematic approach for improving learning, can change a student's attitude by raising self-efficacy, persistence, and a willingness to accept more instruction and new challenges (Arsanow & Meichenbaum, 1979; Jones et al., 1987; Winne, 1985).

How to Teach Self-talk

Before self-talk demonstrations begin, students need to be assured that self-talk is a useful strategy to help themselves learn new skills. It is important for learners to see and hear an expert sample of self-talk applied to a motor skill. Students should have the opportunity to view the skill they will be working on and listen to self-talk about the procedure and how it feels to perform the task, at least twice. A student from the group is then invited to explain how to perform the task. The student gives his/her account of the story and the teacher performs the task. The student must give verbal directions only. Following this presentation, students can work in pairs practicing the task and saying their movement stories out loud so the partner can listen in. On occasion, the teacher should also perform the task incorrectly so students can hear and see how to deal with errors or omissions using self-talk.

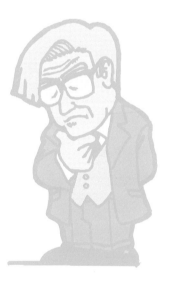

Some children may still experience difficulties. The teacher can then have the students tell their story and pretend to be the performer in order to give them a sense of how powerful the description can be in guiding performance. Students then attempt to clarify and direct the teacher towards successful performance. If this is not effective, the teacher may need to repeat the story from the beginning, as well as the actions that accompany each part of the task. Often students have a sense which part of the action needs help. For example, students may be more inclined to say, "Watch my arm action; it feels funny."

Listen and encourage students to tell themselves exactly what they want to do, to praise themselves, and to ask themselves questions like "What am I supposed to do to get ready?" Occasionally, stop to have the children tell their stories. Often students will elaborate on

Self-talk Intensifies Attention to the Relevant Features of Performance

s		
	encode	
	concentrate	
e	analyze	cognitive
	scan	
l	apply	
f	attribute	
	make judgments	affective
t	exert effort	
a	plan	
	monitor	metacognitive
l	evaluate	
	reflect	
k		

demonstrated versions of the teacher's story and may come to create their own stories to describe movements over time. For example, I asked my 10-year-old daughter to develop a movement story to help her remember how to hold her hands for the volleyball underhand pass. After I showed her the correct way to prepare her hands, she thought the overlapping hands looked like a butterfly and the folded wings (thumbs) created the butterfly's body. Children enjoy composing useful metaphors. Each student may create a different metaphor, but in so doing learners begin to understand that they are largely in control both cognitively and physically of the learning process. Indeed, self talk attempts to shift both the learner's and the teacher's attention away from a single, correct replication of a demonstration to a creative reorganization of a student's own experience in relation to established performance criteria.

Taking ownership for learning is an important step towards enhancing skill acquisition and self-directed learning.

Using the self-talk strategy compels teachers to attend to the learners' agenda. In many cases, teachers are more concerned about what they want students to do, and forgetting how important it is to attend to what the learners are thinking. Teachers typically focus on learners' behaviour, but this can be a misleading source of information about the learners' thought processes and capabilities as self-managers.

Encourage Observation and Analysis   After students have been practicing the proper form for a period of time, challenge students to detect errors on their own. Perform the skill improperly and ask, "What advice would you give a person who performs the trap this way?"

If a learner has difficulty with any aspect of the skill, the teacher should ask the learner to retell the story. If some aspect of the story is omitted the teacher may retell the story and invite the student to select what was missed in his/her story. If difficulties persist, retell the movement story along with a demonstration.

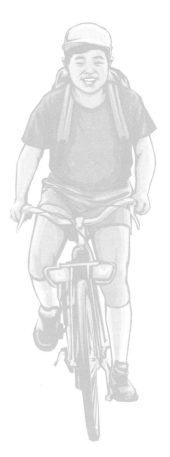

Engaging students in a short discussion about the use of self-talk and then providing them with the script in the form of a friendly dialogue has a settling effect on learners. After hearing an example of the self-talk script, the learner should readily relate to the body action and feel more connected to the task. Skiers focused on the accordion action quickly develop a more rhythmical, merry-go-round, up-and-down action they can enjoy.

Children tend to be natural self-talkers. However, they need to be directed to attend to the important aspects of movement patterns when learning new skills. Again, the self-talk script should be in friendly and familiar terms. Keep the phrases short and let the child fill in the rest of the story. Developmentally delayed children benefit greatly from the use of self-talk. In the following example, Morgan taught me more about the wording (see story in the box, next page).

Although it is necessary to script the action, it is equally important

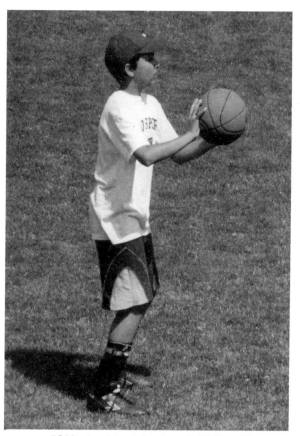

"OK, check out the hands." "Great!"

to be flexible about choosing words learners are more comfortable using. If the learner can supply a word that better matches the body action desired, use it: the choice of words is not set in stone. Children bring a wealth of experience to class and have individual learning styles that will influence the type of words used. Children from other cultures may also draw from different sets of experiences. Sharing them through discussion about the best words, phrases, and metaphors to use for self-talk can open our minds to alternative ways of seeing and thinking.

Guiding Principles of Instructional Self-Talk

Self talk is not a chant Self-talk should be relevant to the understanding of a skill; it is not a meaningless formula to be recited by rote.

Self talk may go underground As skills improve, certain motions become automatic. However, teachers should continue to elicit reaction, analysis, and discussion throughout the development of a skill (e. g., "Tell me what you say to yourself to remember how to catch. Pretend I know nothing about catching. Explain how I should catch").

Morgan's Story

I was teaching the instep kick to a developmentally delayed youngster. To prompt placing his non-kicking foot beside the ball as he kicked, I wanted him to say to himself "step." Morgan prepared to kick the ball and then hesitated because he forgot the word. As his momentum took him forward he said, "walk."

For Morgan, the word "walk" made more sense than "step." In Morgan's mind, stepping is what people do when they climb a flight of stairs. Morgan's image of the movement was better described as a 'walk.' In my workshops, I now encourage young learners to say "walk" to prompt the step action.

Story of a Novice Skier

The movements of beginner skiers tend to be mechanical and rigid. Novices also tend to be overly conscious of other skiers and the terrain before them, which may prevent them from recalling and processing information fast enough to deal with perceived obstacles. Turns and stops seem to come at them in a flurry. Instruction that is focused on the legs and the body opening and closing "like an accordion" prompts a more relaxed and gradual knee flexion and extension. Metaphors learners can relate to help create bridges between new and existing knowledge and experiences. One self-talk script an instructor might use would be: "I start with the accordion closed. As I approach the turn I begin to open the accordion slowly, lean downhill towards the tips of the skis, and then begin to close the accordion as I come through the turn." Repeat the demonstration accompanied by self-talk. Instruct the students to replicate not only the body action but also the instructional script. Encourage students to say the script out loud. Skiers can talk themselves through the movements before and during each practice run. Instructors can thus 'hear' the students thinking and track whether students have the correct sense of what to do both cognitively and physically.

Teachers must know the performance criteria they wish to apply to a skill They should study the description and analysis of movement textbooks and consult physical education specialists for detailed information.

Children cannot use self-talk or any other learning strategy to acquire skills beyond their psychomotor development Students must be physically and mentally ready to learn certain skills. The absence of specific abilities and physical capacity may interfere with involvement and the development of a skill, although modified versions of the mature form of the same skill may facilitate learning.

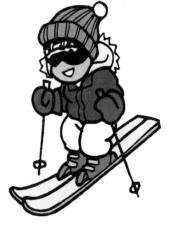

Encourage children to share their stories with each other They can keep journals to describe how they perform a given skill, and to record their ideas about self-talk.

Build a repertoire of metaphors and movement language Brainstorm lists of vivid and expressive language that students can

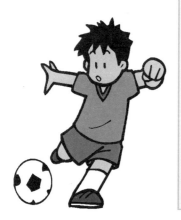

A Self-talk Sequence for Trapping a Soccer Ball

General Statement:

"Do you remember last day what we said we should say to remember to trap the ball?"

Specific Statements:

"Eyes on the ball, get behind the ball, cushion with my big foot (wide part of the foot). Make the trap soft and quiet like a catch. OK, I know what to do – let's try it."

---

draw on to explain their actions.

Listen to what children say to, and about, themselves Encourage students to articulate and communicate their thinking. Students should come to realize that analyzing their thinking is an important part of the learning process.

Be a good model Use self-talk and think aloud regularly to let students in on your thinking. Children need to know that planning for activity is not an impulsive or intuitive act, but the product of careful, logical thought processes.

Handouts and Workshop Activities for Students

The handouts found in the appendix should be distributed to the students and discussed.

"Do you ever talk to yourself?" "Why?" "When?" "Have you ever heard other people talk or say things to themselves?"

On chart paper make a list of occasions when students have used or overheard self-talk being used. Discuss the purpose of self-talk in these situations (e.g., to block out distractions, improve focus etc.).

Begin a list that identifies the key features of a good self-talker (e.g., good self-talkers are positive, use picture words, focus on quality, practice often, etc.).

When Developing Self-talk as a Learning Strategy:

1. Inform students that self talk is natural and can help them remember and concentrate on the task.

2. Break the skill into components or steps where necessary.

3. Collaborate on developing a movement story using cue words, metaphors, or analogies to help students connect novel tasks with familiar actions.

4. Model the action in combination with the movement story or self-talk cue words.

5. Let students also instruct you as teacher.

6. Encourage students to perform a skill using self-talk. Suggest they become their own teachers by telling their body parts what to do and to think. Urge them to use self-talk aloud so you and the others can listen to the dialogue.

7. Praise the use of the strategy: "I like the way you are telling your feet to get ready before you start the throw."

8. Discuss what students are thinking about: "What do you tell yourself when getting ready to throw?"

9. Probe students about their understanding of the task requirements: "What should your arm look like when you throw the ball?" "What could you say to yourself to help you remember to keep your arm bent?"

10. Determine what the student finds difficult - "What part of the skill do you still find confusing?" "What goes through your mind as you are practicing?"

11. Encourage students to articulate their thoughts and actions clearly: "You be my teacher; tell me what I'm supposed to do to throw the ball properly."

12. Talk to students about what they think about using the self-talk strategy.

13. Challenge the students to find other occasions where they can use self-talk.

Distribution of the workshop sheets will vary depending on the number of classes per week and the age of the learners. Some teachers may find certain activities too advanced for younger students. Ideally, the use of self-talk should span the entire school experience, starting in the primary years and reaching routine use by adolescence. Continued use will depend on the teacher's commitment to self-regulated learning, the time available, and the degree to which students are able to grasp the relevant concepts. Self-talk comes only after students have become comfortable using picture words, have explored and experienced imagery, and feel ready to apply a third strategy to their learning.

Self-talk Summary

Our inner voice is a constant companion. Conversations with ourselves remind us what and how to do things. Learning is a social experience. Self-talk is a dimension of the social interaction we have with others as we interact with experiences and others. Self-talk like imagery can be scripted and carefully constructed to ensure we say the 'right' thing to improve performance. Self-talk should be positive, focused on performance enhancement. Self-talk should facilitate learning, hence the use of picture words to add meaning. Self-talk should be friendly, affirming, confident, and focused on key elements of high quality performance. Self-talk is a normal part of everyday life. Used routinely and deliberately, self-talk can be a powerful way to guide learning, analyze movement, and direct attention.

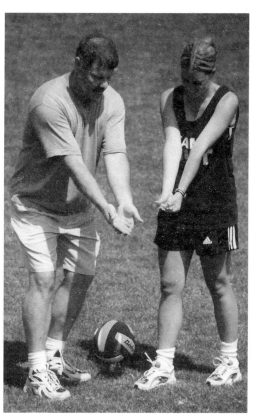

Teachers and students can create a self-talk script together.

Building Understanding

♦ Survey others to find out what they say to themselves in various situations:

a) learning a new skill
b) when threatened
c) to build confidence
d) to cope with stress

♦ What does the use of self-talk seem to suggest about the learning process?

♦ How can self-talk be incorporated into daily routines for learning in class/ out of class?

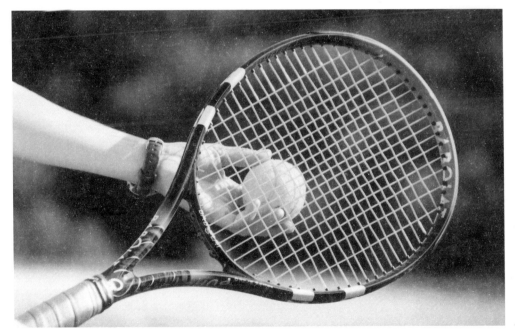

What do you tell yourself when getting ready to serve?

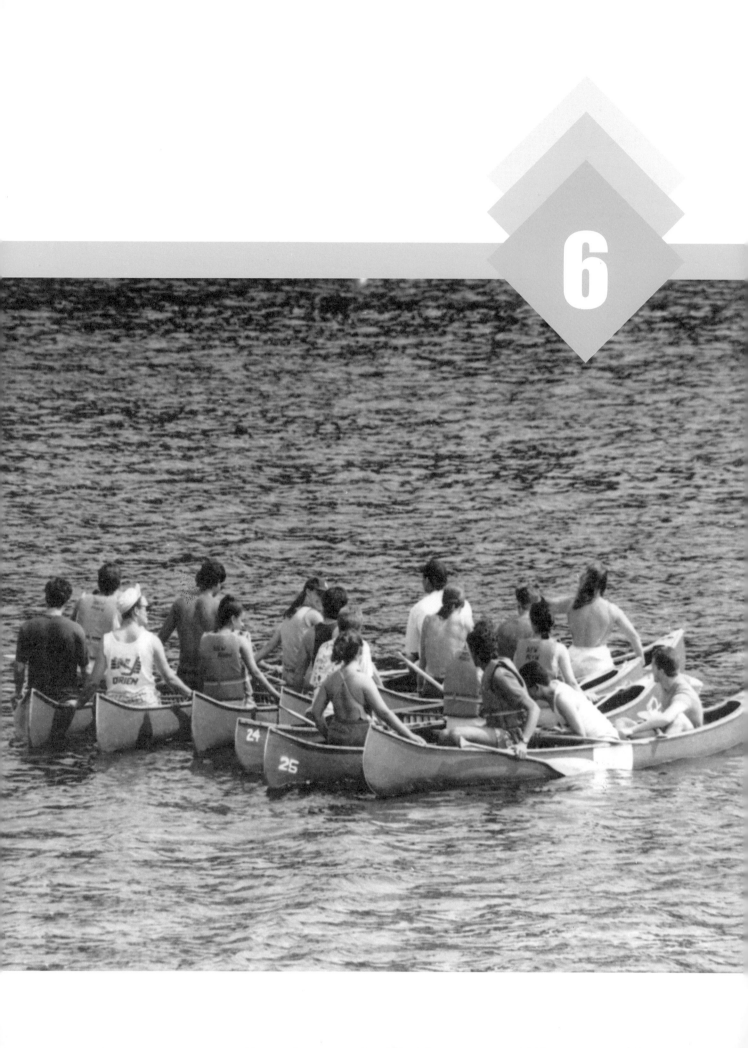

6

GOAL-SETTING

Chapter Outline

- ◆ Definition of Goal–setting

- ◆ Goal Orientations

- ◆ Criteria for Setting Goals

- ◆ How to Teach Goal-setting

- ◆ An Example of Process-oriented Goals

- ◆ Factors to Consider When Goal-setting

- ◆ S.M.A.R.T. Principle

- ◆ Handouts and Workshop Activities for Students

Chapter Objectives

Identify components of an effective goal-setting strategy

Relate goal-setting to learning and skill improvement

Use the S.M.A.R.T. principle to help students set and maintain goals for learning

Teach students how to set, revise, maintain goals for learning

Use classroom ready materials to build goal-setting skills

"Am I on the right road?"
asks the frustrated traveller.

"Depends on where you want to go!"
replies the gas station attendant.

Students achieve more when it is clear what they are expected to do, when they understand the purpose of the activity, and when they know what the end result will be. In other words, students want to know the goals they should set for themselves. Goal-setting is one way learners can sharpen their understanding of a skill or activity and plan its progress. Learners with goals are often more determined and focused than learners who are simply going through the motions. Learning about the goal-setting process and the strategies goal-setters use is an important life skill. This next section explores goal-setting as a learning strategy and explores ways other strategies presented in this book can be incorporated into goal-setting.

Definition of Goal-setting

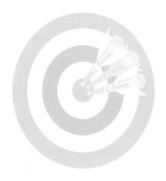

Goals are what an individual tries to accomplish. Goal selection and refinement should be a methodical, deliberate process constructed in response to a careful assessment of needs, aspirations, and abilities. Like most learning strategies, goal-setting should ultimately enable learners to set and monitor their own development and achievement, and thus become more self-reliant and resourceful about their progress.

Goal Orientations

According to Burton (1992), every goal has two basic components: direction and quantity. Direction refers to the focus of the goal for an individual (the score board, elements of form, strategy use). Quantity refers to the amount or minimal standard of performance the individual is willing to accept as a measure of success (70% accuracy, defeat an opponent, achieve a personal best). Direction and quantity interact to produce three distinct goal orientations.

Process-oriented goals are focused on the elements needed to learn the skills and to improve an individual's performance (e.g., "I need to work on getting my racquet back early to prepare for the forehand swing"), not on demonstrating his/her ability to others. My (performance-oriented) goal for the next three practice sessions is to get my racquet back early. To help me remember do this while I am playing, I am going to use self-talk, "racquet back early."

Success-oriented goals are aimed at competitive outcomes and positive social comparisons. For example, "I really want to beat Jeff in tennis. Jeff has always been the best, so until I can beat Jeff, I will not be happy with my tennis skills. I know I can beat Jeff if I keep the game intense by making him run and hurry his swing."

Goal orientations significantly influence a learner's perceptions of ability, effort, persistence in the face of failure, strategy use, self-efficacy, and commitment over time (Burton, 1992; Locke & Latham, 1985). Unless guided to use goal-setting techniques to focus on the steps that lead to skill development, many youngsters may inadvertently sabotage their efforts to try new skills and improve upon existing talents.

Criteria for Setting Goals

Goals are instrumental in the development of skills in two ways. First, goals are concerted efforts on the part of the performer to accomplish a specific task. Goal-setting forces performers to analyze the demands of the task and to accomplishing it through focused, diligent, persistent effort, and the use of appropriate learning strategies such as picture words, imagery, and self-talk. In addition to taking specific physical steps towards improvement, it is important to work on the mental aspects of performance as well. Developing strong imagery skills may be just as important as physical fitness and fine motor control. Second, goals contribute to the performer's perceptions of his/her ability to accomplish tasks. Goal-setting and goal achievement combine to establish an "I can" attitude towards challenges. Goals, therefore, have a stress management role. Setting short-term, well-defined, realistic, performance-oriented goals towards which the learner can work progressively fosters effort and persistence, reduces the anxiety of potential failure, and encourages the use of strategies to overcome barriers.

How to Teach Goal-setting

Plans are stepping stones to achievement that can themselves become measures of performance. Selecting appropriate goals requires thought and care. Organize and write out the plan. Break larger tasks into their smaller, more manageable components through skill analysis. Decide (a) which aspects of a skill need practice and (b) what sort of mental preparation will best foster concentration and eventual success. The planning process shows students how mature learners systematically and methodically address goal attainment.

Begin by setting goals for the class as a whole, such as changing for physical education class in less than 5 minutes. In this example, the process of setting goals and the strategies used to achieve them can be studied collectively and in isolation from those factors (emotional, social, physical) that impinge on individual goal-setting. Together, students can discuss what they need to do to achieve the goal (check before class to make sure gym clothes are ready; not talk too much in the change room; help each other tie shoes, etc.) Care must be taken to focus the attention of students on actions that generate a specific result. The teacher can monitor achievement and recognize progress through individual and collective feedback.

Each lesson should target a specific outcome. Teachers should make clear how lesson activities are related to the overall and intermediary goals of the program. Each skill taught in class should be presented in a way that reveals its component parts as well as the thinking process that underlies it. A balance beam example is shown in the box.

An Example of Process-oriented Goals

A teacher has worked hard to eliminate situations that could interfere or contradict the messages about learning and practice he felt were important. During a basketball lesson, for example, he had taped a number of Xs on the floor that were within three to four metres of the basket. No one was allowed to shoot outside the Xs.

Why? The students' shot mechanics deteriorated outside the four-metre distance. Eager to make three-point shots like the pros, stu-

Goals for learners should be:

Realistic: set goals that are physically achievable.

Specific: identify the behaviours and mental strategies that enable the outcomes to be achieved (to improve my tennis game I will track the ball like a laser beam all the way into my racquet; I will practice imagining tracking the ball all the way to my racquet).

Vivid: if possible detail the goal in terms that enable the performer to see it, feel it, hear it ("My catching goals are to make my catches quiet and soft.").

Realizable in the short-term: unless some measure of success occurs within the first few tries, children often declare themselves inadequate, "I'm no good at this." Youngsters relate and respond better to goals that are achievable within minutes of practice versus days and weeks of practice.

Linked to some plan of action or strategy: attach other strategies such as self-talk to goal attainment, along with a fitness training program that will enhance performance relative to the immediate goals (I need to improve my flexibility in order to do better walkovers; therefore, my goal is to work daily on these two shoulder stretching exercises).

Suited to progressive levels of attainment: achieve competency in form before functional and contextual competency.

Positive: setting positive goals promotes intrinsic motivation and rewards. Think constructively rather than negatively; you will feel better about yourself even when you make mistakes.

Associated with some long-term aspiration: effective educators show students the larger purpose to which all goals must be related. "What's this good for?", a common question among students, in fact signals their need to know how the piece of the puzzle they are working on today fits into the overall picture. Charts that relate, for example, fundamental movement skills such as throwing and catching to lifelong active living pursuits, endow specific goals with significance. Brief, anticipatory discussions before skills are introduced and others after the lesson, summarizing the main points, are opportune times to connect the topic of the lesson with advanced skill attainment (skills, like houses, are built from the foundation up, and according to a well designed set of plans).

dents sacrificed technique for power, hurling the ball through the air, risking injury to others and wasting time needed to develop proper

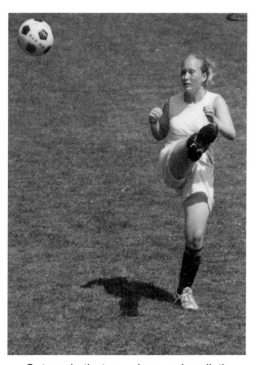

Set goals that are clear and realistic.

form. A significant portion of each class was devoted to shot mastery. Students stood across from each other (about three meters apart) and performed the set shot back and forth. Each partner was expected to make comments about the elements of form they noticed in the shot. The teacher had made and displayed a chart showing the keys to successful shooting, with cue words to describe the elements of form desired ('goose neck' referred to the way the wrist was snapped during the shot to create back spin on the ball). This drill was repeated every class for about two minutes. The teacher emphasized how this drill would help the students improve their shots and their ability to analyze the shot for themselves and their peers. Time was devoted during this drill to offering one-on-one advice and reinforcing the peer feedback process.

How You Do It

When learning to walk on the balance beam, a teacher might ask students to think about the stages a newborn colt goes through when learning to walk: first the colt stands on wobbly legs, often leaning against its mother; then it stands by itself; next, it tries to take a step or two. Learning to walk across the balance beam is a lot like a newborn colt's experience.

Teacher: "We want to include locomotor movements in a routine on the balance beam, while displaying correct form, confidence, and safety: what would be our first set of goals?"

Student: "Stand up on the beam."

Teacher: " Yes, it would be to be able to stand on the beam. Today we will be working on different standing positions on the beam."

Display a list of the standing positions (preferably in pictorial form) and how they can be incorporated into beam routines. Emphasize the importance of balance in a range of activities such as dance, skiing, snowboarding, and sail boarding. At the end of class, refer to a list of goals (travel competently, confidently, and safely along the beam), sub-goals (stand on one foot, stand in a straddle position sideways, etc.), and strategies (for better balance, look at a spot on the beam).

Mary's Short- and Long-term Goals

In the story below, Mary has begun to develop process-oriented goals. Identify the strategies she uses and the effect they have on her progress. Mary is a 12-year-old who loves to play basketball. Although Mary misses more shots than she makes, the mechanics of her set shot continue to improve. She frequently solicits the advice of her teacher, asking questions about her footwork, arm action, and picture words she can use to improve her technique. Outside class, Mary practices with her father in the driveway at home playing one-on-one games. With the help of her teacher Mary has created a set of self-talk words that are related to the key elements of the set shot that she says aloud to herself as she takes a shot: "Knees, platform, rim, goose neck into the hoop." Occasionally, she shares her self-talk words with other students. She willingly accepts feedback and is excited by the challenges the game offers.

Mary's short-term goals are to perfect the mechanics of the set shot; specifically, hand placement on the ball, arm action, body position, and use of the legs in shooting. In the back of Mary's mind there are two long term goals; one is to shoot with picture-perfect form during game play; the other is to beat her dad in a game of 21.

At predetermined intervals, the teacher evaluated the students. The first evaluation was a self-evaluation. Each student was given a check sheet (see sample). The students could take four shots at their own pace, from anywhere on the court. Two points were awarded for each element of form correctly executed at this stage of development. One point was given for putting the ball through the hoop.

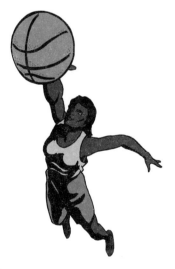

The second evaluation was assigned for homework. Each student was given the necessary materials to make a drawing or plasticine figure of a player preparing for a set shot. The caption below the figurine was expected to display the principal elements of form.

The third evaluation consisted of a short video clip of a shot with poor technique. Each student was required to give three pieces of strategic advice to the player in the video, two about the player's form and the third about how the player could improve his or her performance.

The final evaluation involved videotaping each child's set shot. A drill was set up that involved approaching the basket, receiving a

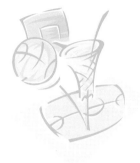

pass, and shooting. Each student was allowed two attempts. The student's technique was evaluated on a five-point scale consisting of the five key elements of form displayed in class (see below).

Factors to Consider When Goal-setting

Three factors have a bearing on goal-setting used to advance performance: situation, goal commitment, and feedback.

Situation   In practice situations, the emphasis is generally on learning and skill improvement. Social pressure is lower and the motivational function of goals can play a significantly positive role. Goals are more likely to be process-oriented, focusing on the purpose of the skill and building the intensity and range of applications of particular moves. For example, during gymnastic classes, students learn the fundamentals of the forward roll and then are gradually introduced to a variety of ways to start, finish, and connect the forward roll to other gymnastic moves and poses. Learners can also begin to explore different levels, directions, and relationships with equipment and partners (rolling down an incline, performing forward rolls simultaneously with a partner, etc.)

Good shooters face the hoop and remember the five important points.

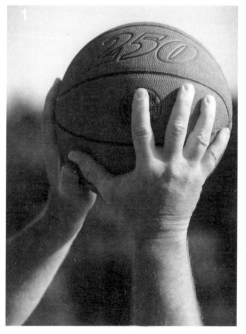

"J"
(index finger and thumb form a 'J')

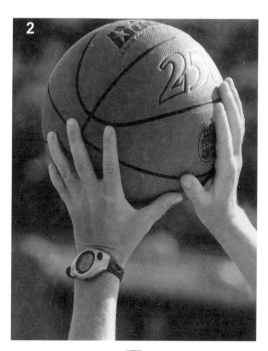

"T"
(thumbs make a 'T')

Basketball Set Shot Evaluation Form

Student's Name: _____   **Age:** _____

Good shooters remember to:

	--	-	0	+	++
"J"	____	____	____	____	____
"T"	____	____	____	____	____
"V"	____	____	____	____	____
"Z"	____	____	____	____	____
Goose neck	____	____	____	____	____

By contrast, the competitive situation invites social comparison and places a greater emphasis on achievement. Goals are likely to

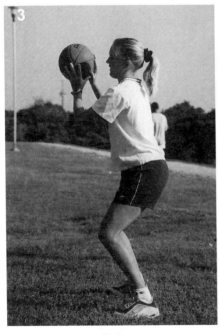

"V"
(elbows are bent)

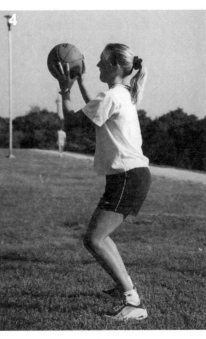

"Z"
(knees bent—body forms a 'Z')

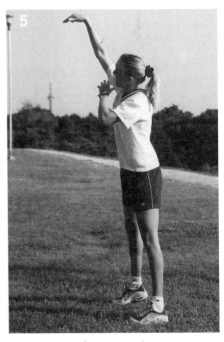

Goose neck

become more success- and failure-oriented, making stress management more important. Here, goals should emphasize poise, mental toughness, and optimal performance through concentration and diligence.

Goal commitment   The goal-setting process is influenced by the commitment learners make to the goal, which is markedly different for each goal-setting orientation. Process-oriented participants base their commitment primarily on intrinsic factors (enhanced sense of self and sense of efficacy), whereas performers oriented towards success or failure rely on extrinsic factors (trophies, praise) to support their efforts. Process-oriented learners will maintain allegiance to any goal that will help them learn or improve a skill. Success-oriented learners will maintain their commitment only as long as they appear to be doing well in comparison with others. Failure-oriented individuals are unlikely to commit to any competitive goal for fear of embarrassment.

Feedback   Feedback should promote goal-setting for both process-oriented and success-oriented performers, but impairs failure-oriented performers. For the process- and success-oriented students, positive feedback confirms that learning and improvement are occurring. Negative feedback signals the need to adjust the strategies used or to increase effort. Feedback for the failure-oriented further impairs performance because success is attributed largely to uncontrollable factors such as luck. Even positive feedback is ineffective because it makes negative social comparison more explicit. For example, a novice skier was praised for keeping her skis parallel during the turn. The failure-oriented learner dismissed the praise. "I got lucky that time, I won't be able to do that again. I'm such a klutz compared to the rest of the group."

Process-oriented goals are preferable, especially during the early stages of skill development. If young learners can begin by thinking about what it takes to improve the form of their skills and the strategies that enable them to concentrate and to persist in practice, a greater number of children and adolescents will gain personal and social satisfaction as well as health benefits from involvement in physical education programs and remain committed to physical activity throughout life.

Milestones

Along the journey to your goals there are significant smaller achievements called milestones. For example, in learning to shoot well, a significant milestone involves positioning the hands on the ball the right way, all the time. In other words, making this part of the skill a habit or routine. Once it is a habit, your mind is free to concentrate on other aspects of performance such as bending the knees ("Z position").

In the goal planning sheet provided, list the milestones that will enable you to achieve your goal.

S.M.A.R.T. Principle

Good goal-setters are smart. They use the S.M.A.R.T. principle.

S: Make your goal *specific*. Rather than saying, "I'll improve abdominal strength," state, "I'm going to do 3 sets of 20 curl ups on Monday, Thursday, and Saturday."

M: Make your goal *measurable*. Can you see whether or not you have achieved your goal? " Yes, I completed 3 sets of 20 repetitions on Monday, Thursday, and Saturday."

A: Make your goal *attainable*. Commit to small, short term challenges. "Today I'll take the stairs instead of the elevator."

R: Make your goal *realistic*. Be flexible. Set a goal that will fit into your lifestyle and schedule. "I'll take a stretch break at 10:00 each morning, that doesn't interfere with anything."

T: Give yourself a *time limit*. Set a time when you will look back to see if you have met your goal: "I will review my plans in three weeks."

Handouts and Workshop Activities for Students

Use the worksheets to guide home study and further discussions in class. It is important that students engage in independent study to

Benefits of goal-setting:

♦ clarifies direction

♦ organizes strategy use

♦ maintains focus on specific targets

♦ focuses practice

♦ builds motivation

Goal Planning Sheet

Student's Name: _____   **Age:** _____

Long-term Goal:

_____

_____

Projected Date of Achievement:

_____

Milestone #1:

_____

_____

Date:

_____

Milestone #2:

_____

_____

Date:

_____

Milestone #3:

_____

_____

Date:

_____

learn how goal-setting is used to guide and improve performance. Throughout the process teachers need to touch base with students individually or collectively to share ideas, make revisions, and reorganize

Good Goal-setters:

♦ commit to working on goals every day

♦ set goals every day so they learn how to be good goal-setters

♦ image their goal: see, feel, and hear the results every day

♦ simulate or run through what they have to do in practice.

♦ re-evaluate goals after practices and run-throughs (it's OK to make changes)

♦ are totally connected to their task in mind and body

♦ use self-talk to direct their actions

♦ are persistent, knowing that learning to be a good goal-setter takes time

♦ celebrate their achievements: smile inside and out

♦ focus 100% every step of the way during run-throughs

plans. Students need to understand that goal-setting is a careful plan aimed at improvements in the qualitative aspects of performance. There are many external variables, the internal variables – self confidence, focus on key elements of quality performance – are variables students can control from the 'inside'.

The worksheets can be distributed to all students. Take time to discuss use of the sheets so students understand that it can take several days to think through their plans. It is best to incorporate goal-setting as 'core' material. In other words, goal-setting is not an 'add on.' It is a life-skill that, if used appropriately, can make an important difference in any area of study.

Students may not have the time to perfect skills in class; therefore, it is important they use learning plans and goals to support home study. Students realize how much they can do on their own and the significance of strategy use to promote self-directed and self-reliant learning.

Good goal-setters are smart. They use the S.M.A.R.T. principle.

Goal-setting Summary

Characteristics of Effective Goals:

- realistic
- specific
- vivid
- near-sighted
- linked to strategies
- personalized
- suitable
- associated with long term aspirations

Characteristics of Goals:

- focus
- direction

Goal Orientations:

- process-oriented goals
- success-oriented goals
- failure-oriented goals

Set attainable goals.

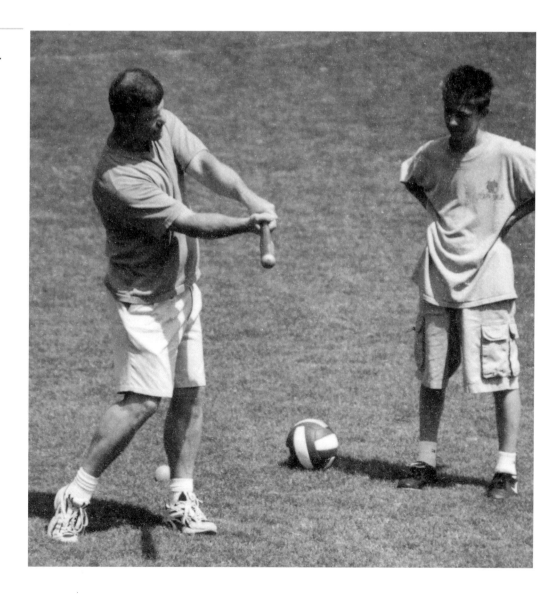

Building Understanding

♦ Interview adults to find out how they use goal-setting in their lives: work, home, family life. Make a list of the different ways goal-setting influences daily life.

♦ Can you find any quotes about goals?

♦ Read or listen to interviews with high performance athletes to find out if they set goals.

♦ Keep a journal of the goals you set for skill improvement within this class. Can you develop a graph to depict changes in your performance?

♦ Interview a coach to find out more about goal-setting. Ask: What are your team goals? What goals do players on your team set?

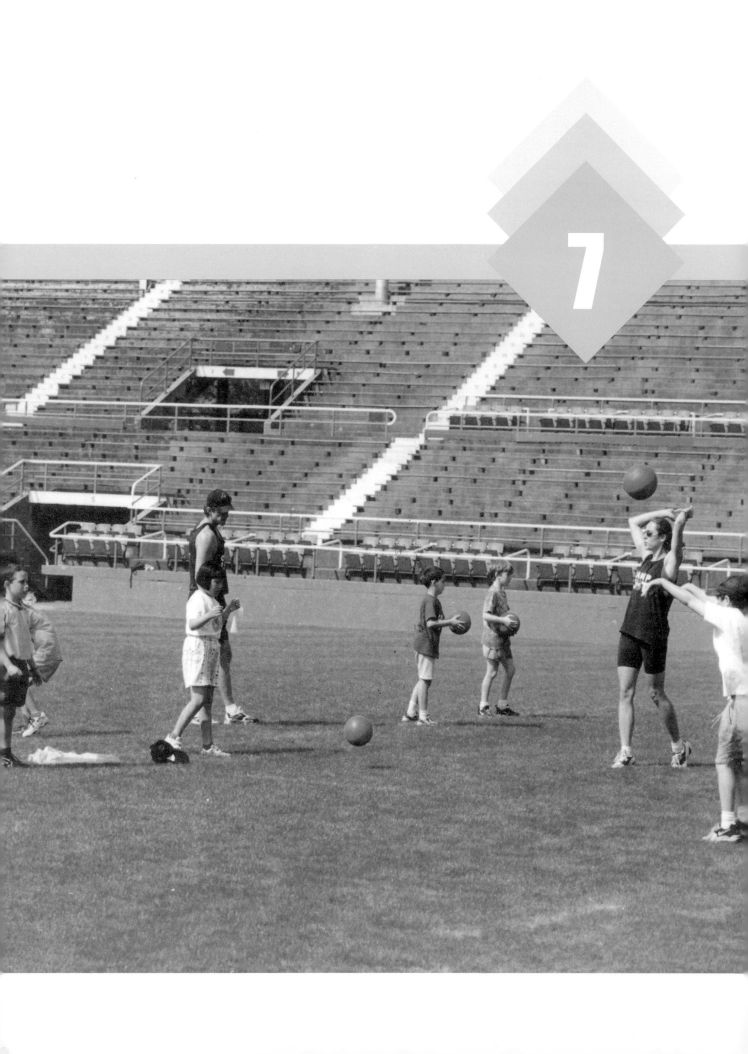

7

ASSESSMENT AND EVALUATION

Chapter Outline	Chapter Objectives
♦ Basic Literacy	Distinguish between basic, critical, and dynamic literacy
♦ Critical Literacy	
♦ Dynamic Literacy	Use indicators to assess strategy use and proficiency
♦ Stages of Development	
	Relate stages of development to strategy use and self-reliant learning
	Use assessment as an integral part of the teaching/learning process

Assessment and evaluation should be an integral part of the teaching and learning process.

Assessment and evaluation should be an integral part of the teaching and learning process (Anderson & Goode, 1997). Woven into instruction and self-management, assessment enables learners to track progress and make adjustments, evaluate progress, and realign preparation and performances with the goals. The first step in effective assessment and evaluation

is establishing clear, relevant, and realistic goals. Too often, beginners set out to play on all-star teams, become professional athletes, or break records. Although inspiring, these goals are too distant and do little to enhance the planning that is necessary to achieve the desired results. Helping learners set, plan, and monitor the achievement of skills that are within their grasp is both rewarding and motivating.

Three forms of 'literacy' pertaining to learning strategy use are addressed below: basic, critical, and dynamic.

Basic Literacy

**Benefits of as-
sessment and
evaluation:**

♦ Provides informa-
tion to both stu-
dents and teach-
ers

♦ A resource for de-
cision-making

♦ Facilitates plan-
ning

♦ Defines learning
expectations

♦ Enables teachers
to coordinate in-
struction with
outcomes

♦ Enables students
to set their sites
on both process
and product

In basic literacy, the learner is able to distinguish among the different kinds of strategies, describe what is involved in their use, and identify how strategies facilitate learning. Questions the learner can answer include: What are the characteristics of the strategy? What does it look like, sound like, feel like? What are you supposed to be able to do with picture words (imagery, self-talk, goal-setting)? How do these techniques improve learning and skill development? When should you use them? What are the benefits of using them?

Critical Literacy

In critical literacy, the learner can analyze, interpret and explain whether, which, and under what conditions particular learning strategies are appropriate. Questions the learner can address include: Which learning strategy will help me learn better? How should I use this particular learning strategy to learn better? What key elements of performance should I be concentrating on?

Dynamic Literacy

In dynamic literacy, the learner is able to manage strategy use confidently and independently and on a regular basis and in accordance with the demands of the skill and the situation (strategy use is deliberate, routine, and embedded in skill performance). The learner personalizes the use of a particular strategy or combinations of strategies and is will-

Indicators of Basic Achievement

Self-evaluation

I Can

	yes	almost
♦ recognize particular kinds of strategies	☐	☐
♦ use common names for each strategy	☐	☐
♦ describe key elements of strategy use	☐	☐
(picture words contain images that are familiar)		
♦ describe how I use particular strategies	☐	☐

Teacher Evaluation

_____ **can**
(student's name)

	yes	almost
♦ recognize particular strategies	☐	☐
♦ use common names for each strategy	☐	☐
♦ describe key elements of strategy use	☐	☐
♦ describe how s/he uses particular strategies	☐	☐

ing to be flexible and to adapt them. In both the performance of skills and other areas of life, learning strategy use has become commonplace.

This process may take several years, but eventually, the dynamic learner recognizes how to use particular learning strategies to enhance learning in almost any situation. The strategic learner has moved from clearing obstacles to trying to obtain a deeper understanding of how specific movements are performed, how existing movement skills are related to developing new skills, how to manage cognitive and metacognitive plans, and how to apply plans to improve game play or conquer personal achievement challenges. In other words, learners have the capacity to be knowledge-builders rather

Indicators of Critical Achievement

Self- Evaluation

I Can

	yes	almost
◆ recognize when strategy use is helpful	☐	☐
◆ explain how to use the strategy appropriately	☐	☐
◆ describe how particular strategies affect learning	☐	☐
◆ detect errors	☐	☐

Teacher Evaluation

_____ **can**

(student's name)

	yes	almost
◆ recognize when strategy use is helpful	☐	☐
◆ explain how to use the strategy appropriately	☐	☐
◆ describe how particular strategies affect learning	☐	☐
◆ detect errors	☐	☐

than just knowledge consumers. Competent knowledge-builders strategically interact with information. Whether or not they have good teachers, they can make the best of the information available. They can also elaborate on their experiences and generate motor and cognitive plans that intensify and augment the learning process. They are self-directed, self-reliant learners.

Stages of Development

Educational Phase

◆learners seek to understand the mechanics of strategy, how, when, and where strategies may be applied (What sorts of words can I use to self-talk? What does talking to yourself look like, sound like? How much

Indicators of Dynamic Achievement

Self- Evaluation

I Can

	yes	almost
♦ select and apply strategies to skill development	☐	☐
♦ make adjustments to the strategy as needed	☐	☐
♦ routinely use strategies to enhance performance	☐	☐
♦ reflect on strategy use	☐	☐

Teacher Evaluation

_____ **can**

(student's name)

	yes	almost
♦ select and apply strategies to skill development	☐	☐
♦ make adjustments to the strategy as needed	☐	☐
♦ routinely use strategies to enhance performance	☐	☐
♦ reflect on strategy use	☐	☐

should I say to myself? How do I know whether I am self-talking appropriately?)

Application Phase

♦ learners approach routine use of strategies

♦ learners co-construct strategy application (helping the teacher develop the imagery or self-talk scripts)

♦ goals, milestones, and ladders to success are negotiated collaboratively

Refinement Phase

♦ learners personalize use of the strategy

♦ learners customize and adjust the use of strategies to meet needs and goals and overcome challenges

♦learners are able to monitor the adequacy of the strategy and make alterations to suit circumstances and progress

Self-directed Learning Phase

♦learners independently select, adapt, and tailor use of various strategies and combinations of strategies to fulfill learning goals

♦learners construct learning strategies according to situations and principles of effective strategy use

♦learners orchestrate their own learning

The evaluation guide presented here (opposite page) offers students and educators a visual representation of the activities associated with progression through the phases of development. Activities on the outer ring are intended to help learners discover more about particular strategy use. As learners progress towards the centre, they are able to demonstrate more control and are expected to use strategies more routinely and as an integral part of the learning process. Symbolically, the closer the learner is to the centre the more focused, cognitively aware, and concentrated his/her efforts are towards learning.

Assessment and Evaluation Summary

Assessment and evaluation involves data collection and judgment-making. Three forms of literacy are at work: basic, critical, and dynamic. At each level, students are encouraged to 'think' about their work – what did I learn? What does this mean? Where do I go from here? Assessment and evaluation should be aimed at both process (how do I get there?) and product (what will I end up with?). Focus on process should predominate because in schools we are preparing students to think more carefully about how they go about learning. Eventually, we hope they will be more resourceful, thoughtful, and strategic learners. However, the only way they really know if learning was successful is when they perform the skills and match them against standards set by the teacher or themselves or both. They need to relate inputs (both good and bad, successful and not so successful) to outcomes (standards, expectations, goals). Assessment and evaluation should be considered before and throughout the learning process.

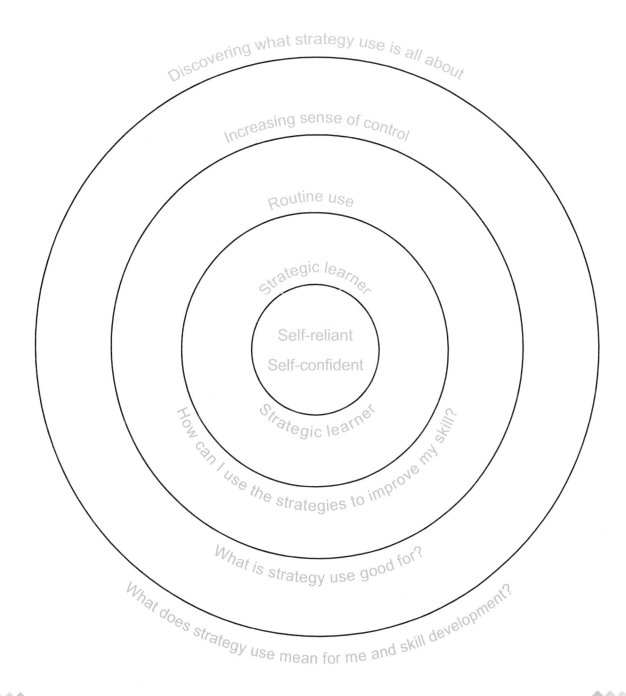

Discovering what strategy use is all about

Increasing sense of control

Routine use

Strategic learner

Self-reliant

Self-confident

Strategic learner

How can I use the strategies to improve my skill?

What is strategy use good for?

What does strategy use mean for me and skill development?

Building Understanding

♦ Develop a report card that emphasizes strategy use.

♦ Invite students to prepare a report card for strategy use.

♦ Prepare task cards for strategy use.

Appendix

Picture Words

The Missing 'Think'

What are picture words?

Can you think of the actions you would perform if you were told to "curl up small like a mouse" or "be as tall as a tree," "swing your arms like an elephant's trunk" or "explode off the base." These are picture words and phrases. Picture words are meaningful and memorable ways to describe how to move.

Here are the picture words for catching a ball:

- Make a spider web or basket with the glove or your hands

- Reach out

- Make the catch quiet/soft like it's landing on a pillow

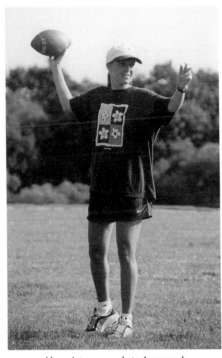

Use picture words to improve!

Benefits of using picture words:

- Remember what to do
- Focus better
- Block out distractions
- Boost confidence
- Boost energy
- Relax
- Improve faster

Special points of interest:

- ♦ Picture words should be friendly
- ♦ Choose pictures that clearly represent the action
- ♦ Practice using the words to direct and check performance
- ♦ Listen to the picture words people use

Kinds of picture words

Seeing words: spread the wings of the eagle

Feeling words: float, glide, strong, punch, cradle

Hearing words: soft, quiet, pillow, crunch

Energizer words: rocket, explode

Relaxing words: soft like marshmallows, float like a leaf

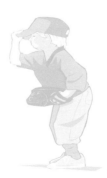

Intensify your practice.

Imagery

What is imagery?

Have you ever heard the expression:

"I can imagine him doing that," or "Picture that in your mind," or

"I just can't picture myself doing this"? What do those expressions tell you?

How many windows are in your home or apartment? What did you do to make the calculation? Before we redecorate a room, organize a party, or prepare for an important interview, we envision or mentally rehearse the performance and the events that lead up to it. It is a perfectly normal way to prepare. It is a way to anticipate, organize, and strategize for the future. Imagery is imagining you are doing the action in your head. Imagery is not just thinking about the movements; it is thinking through the movements in an attempt to realistically replicate the sites, sounds, feelings, and emotions related to the movement experience.

Some people use imagery to cope with stress, for example, when delivering a speech, performing in front of large crowds, dealing with distractions, and improving sports performance. Used properly and appropriately, imagery can be a powerful tool for learning.

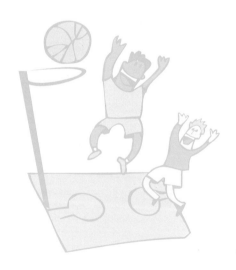

Benefits of using imagery:

- Improve focus
- Block distractions
- Make better plans
- Practice better
- Correct errors
- Calm down
- Review what you are to do

Special points of interest:

♦ Practice imagery often
♦ Apply the skills to different situations
♦ Use all your senses

Prove it to yourself

Take a moment to relax your shoulders, neck, and back. Let your arms and legs become *soft* and *loose*. Let your head balance evenly on your shoulders. Breathe quietly, comfortably, and rhythmically. Now close your eyes and picture yourself in a favourite place with a special person. Picture the scenery. Detail the landscape and the person(s) with you. Feel the contact you are making with the ground, the people, and yourself. Hear the sounds that are around you or are sent to you. Smell the aromas around you. Take a few moments and enjoy the experience and all its sensational effects.

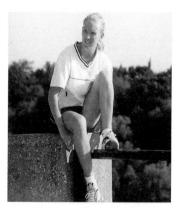

Imagine yourself performing better than ever before.

IMAGERY LEARNING WORKSHOP

IMAGERY AND VIVIDNESS

BENEFITS OF IMAGERY

- Ready mind and body
- Calming, quietening
- Focus attention
- Mental planning
- Improve concentration
- Anticipate problems
- Plan solutions

Special points of interest:

- ■ Practice imagery often
- ■ Practice in a relaxed state
- ■ Use imagery in many ways
- ■ Be positive
- ■ Use imagery to solve problems
- ■ HAVE FUN

Other imagery activities

Imagine:

- ♦ City lights from a hilltop
- ♦ Stars on a clear night
- ♦ A field of flowers
- ♦ The sun as it sinks below the horizon
- ♦ Trees blowing gently in the wind

Workshop focus

This workshop focuses on creating vivid images that you can **see** in your mind.

Before you begin

Make sure your body and your mind are calm and quiet. Imagine yourself floating on a soft fluffy cloud high above the earth, far from troubles and tensions. Let your imagination wander as you enjoy the scenery below and the soft relaxing feeling of floating like a cloud.

Activity

Close your eyes....In your mind's eye see your bedroom. Can you see the bed? Other furniture? Where your clothes are kept? Pictures on the wall? Can you imagine other rooms in your home? Imagine you are taking a person on a guided tour of your home – start at the front door.

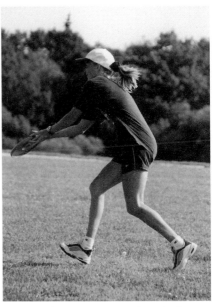

See the frisbee traveling through the air toward your hands. See yourself reach out and make the catch.

USING IMAGERY IN PHYSICAL EDUCATION

Imagine a piece of sports equipment: baseball bat, glove, hockey stick, skates, snowboard. Can you see it clearly? Its shape? Size? Colours? Distinguishing markings? *Close your eyes and imagine the gymnasium space....where is the main entrance (point to it now), imagine the basketball nets on the wall (point to one of them now). Imagine other distinguishing markings or objects in the gym: clock, doors, banners, signs.*

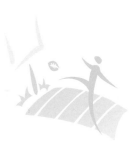

Imagination is powerful.

IMAGERY LEARNING WORKSHOP

IMAGERY AND VIVIDNESS

BENEFITS OF IMAGERY

- Ready mind and body
- Calming, quietening
- Focus attention
- Improve concentration
- Anticipate problems
- Plan solutions

Special points of interest:

- Practice every day
- Practice in a quiet spot
- Develop a routine
- Focus on performance mastery
- Use in everyday living

Other imagery activities

Imagine the feel of:
- cat's fur
- a baby's cheek
- a very tight shoe
- greasy fingers
- sandpaper
- flower petals

Introduction

This workshop focuses on creating vivid images that help you think about the 'feel' of a movement.

Before you begin

Pretend you are an ice cream cone freshly scooped from the container. Now pretend you have been set out in the sun. Feel the warm sun melting you slowly. Continue until all the ice cream is melted.

Activity

Close your eyes. Pretend you are holding/touching a piece of sports equipment: baseball bat, baseball glove, hockey stick, tennis racquet, balance beam. Try to feel its texture, weight, what it is made of, its length, its edges.

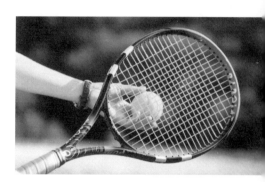
Feel the texture, weight, and 'sweet spot.'

Try it with a racquet in one hand and imagine the other hand holding the same racquet.

USING IMAGERY IN PHYSICAL EDUCATION

Try to see and feel the equipment your are working with in physical education classes or after school clubs/teams. For example; feel the basketball, its texture, weight, grooves, roundness. Sometimes improvements are made when we enhance our *'feel'* for the ground or the apparatus we are working with. Runners imagine the *feel* of the ground beneath them moving smoothly over terrain and varied surfaces. Gymnasts *feel* the balance beam beneath their feet, the shape of the bars, and the texture of the floor exercise mats.

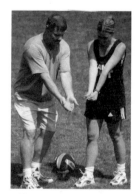
Share imagery stories.

IMAGERY LEARNING WORKSHOP

IMAGERY AND VIVIDNESS

BENEFITS OF IMAGERY

- Get ready for action

- Relax

- Practice without injury

Special points of interest:

■ Practice every day

■ Share your insights with others

■ Be creative

■ Script your actions in your head

Other imagery activities

Imagine sounds:
♦ tennis serve
♦ soccer kick
♦ basketball dribble
♦ underhand pass in volleyball
♦ church bells
♦ rain on a roof
♦ clapping of hands in applause

Introduction

This workshop focuses on creating vivid imagery that helps you think about the sounds of particular movements..

Why is sound imagery important?

The sound the ball makes when it is struck by the batter gives the fielder information about how well the ball was hit. Tennis players know the 'feel' of the sweet spot on the racquet. Gymnasts know the sound of a vault - the running approach, takeoff, punch, flight, and landing. Golfers know the swoosh of an effective swing and the resounding crack of a well-struck ball.

Before you begin

Play soft and soothing music while you imagine a paradise. Imagine the scenery, the plants and animals, and the people you would be with. Listen for the sounds of the wind and the birds.

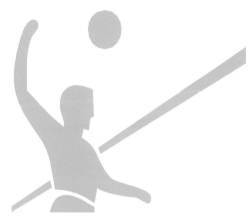

Use imagery to prepare.

Activity

Try to imagine the sounds of a physical activity such as running, skating, swimming, or playing basketball. Listen to the footwork. Can you detect the difference between skipping, galloping and walking? Listen to tiptoeing, marching, and hopping. With a friend, try bouncing some different balls one at a time while s/he closes his or her eyes and listens. Make an audio tape of different movements.

USING IMAGERY IN PHYSICAL EDUCATION

For a skill you are working on, try to listen to the sounds - the environment (pool or gymnasium), the equipment used, other people engaged in the activity, and the distinct action involved (the swoosh of the ball going through the net in basketball). Before practices and in your spare time imagine the game and tune into the sounds of the game, the flow of the body action.

IMAGERY LEARNING WORKSHOP

IMAGERY AND VIVIDNESS

BENEFITS OF IMAGERY

- Re-create the action
- Overcome obstacles
- Rehearse in your head
- Build confidence

Special points of interest:

- Use imagery to organize thoughts and actions
- Ask others how they use imagery

Other imagery activities

Imagine:

- the smell of your favourite foods: chocolate, cheese, pizza
- the smell of your favourite sport : the smell of a swimming pool, tennis court, hockey arena

Introduction

This workshop focuses on imagery related to smell. How much does smell affect feelings and emotions? Imagine the smell of a rose garden, the aroma of a candy store, the taste of a favourite treat.

Before you begin

Think of your body as being uncooked spaghetti - stiff and straight. Now feel your body being slowly immersed in warm water. First your toes become soft and limp, next your ankles, lower legs and thighs. Let your body sink slowly into the water until you are completely immersed. Feel your body become totally relaxed. Think of times in the day when you can do this. What are the benefits?

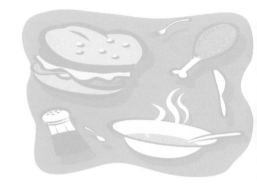

Activity

Pay attention to the smells associated with your skill activity: the smell of chlorine at the pool, the smell of fresh-cut grass at the soccer field, the smell of the autumn air. List them on a sheet of paper. When you image this activity try to image these smells. With a friend , present different pieces of equipment or balls (basketball, tennis ball) and close your eyes. Can you smell the difference?

USING IMAGERY IN PHYSICAL EDUCATION

Smells and tastes are a powerful part of our lives. List three smells and tastes that remind you of important events. Beside each activity list distinct smells:

Basketball, soccer, swimming, cross country skiing, gymnastics, tennis, badminton, floor hockey.

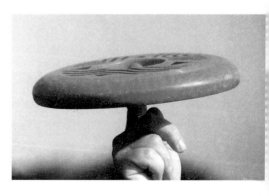

IMAGERY LEARNING WORKSHOP

IMAGERY AND CONTROL

BENEFITS OF IMAGERY

- Polish skills

- Avoid distractions

- Boost confidence

- Challenge yourself

A true story about imagery

One young fellow was afraid of going to the dentist. He decided to imagine his super heroes, Batman and Robin, going to the dentist. They handled the situation in a cool and calm manner. When it came time for the young boy to go to the dentist he imagined his super heroes were with him. It was a success!

Introduction

The next activities focus on imagery for control. Imagery control refers to the ability to manipulate (move, enlarge, rotate, situate) images.

Before you begin

Pretend in your mind that you can travel back in time to any period in history. Imagine you are playing road hockey with players in the 1920's. What if you could visit pioneer days? Imagine introducing the game of basketball to the Knights of the Round Table.

Activity

Stand with your arms at your sides.
Step 1. Imagine you are raising one of your arms from your side to shoulder height.
Step 2. Close your eyes. Imagine raising one

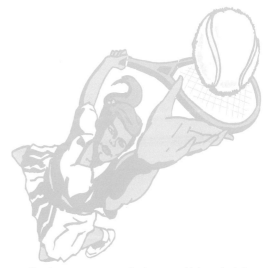

Use imagery to control what you think and do!

of your arms to shoulder height. Repeat steps 1 and 2 using the other arm. Try the same activities again., but pretend you are a spider on the wall watching you raise and lower first your right arm then your left. Observe yourself again but this time be a spider on the ceiling. Tell your partner what it was like doing these activities.

USING IMAGERY IN PHYSICAL EDUCATION

Pretend you are preparing to take turn at bat. Take hold of the bat, feel the weight and texture of the handle. See yourself raising the bat to your shoulder. Observe your stance from different angles. Take a practice swing in your mind. How did it feel? Before you try any activity stop and think it through before you try it. Here are some action phrases to "think" and then "do."

Action Phrases:
Run – freeze – skip
Grow – collapse – pop
Creep – pounce – explode
Chop – whirl – slash
Stretch – slither – crumple
Create your own and let the class try your idea.

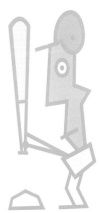

A129

IMAGERY LEARNING WORKSHOP

IMAGERY AND CONTROL

BENEFITS OF IMAGERY

- Control emotions
- Calm nerves
- Stay alert
- Improve skills
- Prepare better

Good imagery users

Good imagery users create images of themselves successfully performing the skill. Try to see yourself doing the 'right' things and making all the 'right' moves. Hear the people around you praising your success. Feel your equipment working perfectly.

Everyday imagery

The next time you have to stand in line for something practice your imagery skills. Make the people in front of you change shape, size, or kind of clothing they are wearing. See how time flies.

Introduction

This workshop focuses on seeing yourself perform various movements from different vantage points.

Before you begin

Imagine you are working the controls of a big screen TV. As you are surfing the channels you come to a station that takes you to a place that is so relaxing and inviting you can't switch the station. Lay back and enjoy the scenery as the program unfolds.

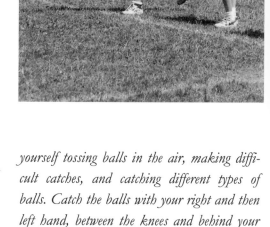

Activity

Imagine you are walking around in your home. In your mind watch this action as if you were on the ceiling looking down at the activity. Now try the activity again but watch from the floor as if you were an ant. Find other spots in the room from which you could observe yourself performing the task. Observe *yourself tossing balls in the air, making difficult catches, and catching different types of balls. Catch the balls with your right and then left hand, between the knees and behind your back, toss and clap your hands before you catch. What an amazing catcher!*

USING IMAGERY IN PHYSICAL EDUCATION

Try the same activity with a sport skill. For example, imagine yourself skating. Position yourself high in the stands watching the activity. Next, pretend you are the blue line watching you skate over and by you. Imagine yourself as the hockey stick or riding on the top of your helmet. What do you see differently?

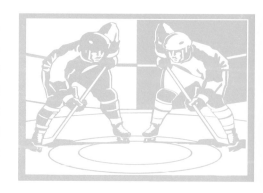

IMAGERY LEARNING WORKSHOP

IMAGERY AND CONTROL

BENEFITS OF IMAGERY

- Feel the action
- Plan for success
- Activity rehearsal
- Improve skills

Special points of interest:

- ◆ Visualization is reality in the mind's eye
- ◆ If you see yourself as a kitten can you change yourself into a tiger?
- ◆ Imagery can be used to see what it is like to be a different person

Introduction

This workshop focuses on *feeling* the movement.

Before you begin

Imagine that you have just put your foot in a bucket of ice water. Can you feel the ice cubes floating around? Now, with the warmth of your imagination, feel yourself melting the ice cubes. Can you feel the tingling? What other sensations are you feeling?

Activity

Raise your arm to your shoulder. Try to feel the action. Now close your eyes and imagine the action and the FEEL of raising your arm. Repeat this activity with different body parts.

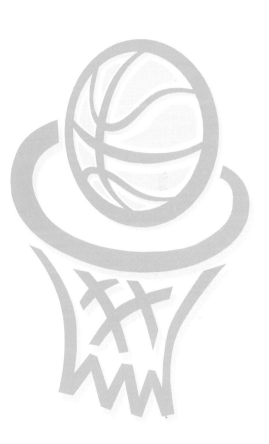

USING IMAGERY IN PHYSICAL EDUCATION

Perform a sport skill such as a tennis swing or wrist shot in hockey. As you perform the skill, try to FEEL the action. Closing your eyes may help. Now try to imagine the action and the feel. Try shooting hoops at a basket with your eyes closed. Talk about what you learned with a friend. Try a somersault with your eyes closed. Feel the mat with your hands, then your upper back through to your seat, then your feet. Try to use the feeling of the movement to improve the smoothness of the action.

IMAGERY LEARNING WORKSHOP

IMAGERY AND CONTROL

- Warm up the mind
- Control emotions
- Plan ahead
- Build confidence
- Correct errors

Special points of interest:

♦ Practice often

♦ Share ideas about imagery with others

♦ Always relax before you begin to image

♦ Use imagery to solve problems

♦ Use imagery to fade out distractions the way a painter brushes out mistakes on the canvas

Introduction

This activity focuses on imaging different body positions.

Before you begin

Imagine being a leaf floating down a beautiful shaded brook. Hear the water trickle over the rocks. Feel yourself being carried along, swirling and gliding. Look up and see the trees, flowers and the bushes go by.

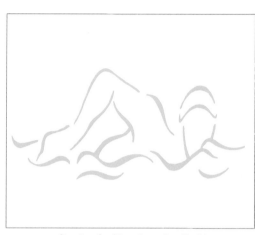

See it – feel it – hear it – Do it!

Activity

Note what it looks and feels like to be seated, standing, lying down, crouched, twisted, and stretched out. Repeat each position several times until you have a strong sense of the position of your body - where your head is, where your arms are, and where your tummy is. Now close your eyes and imagine being seated, standing, lying down, curled into a ball, stretching as if you just got up from sleeping, and twisting into a pretzel shape.

USING IMAGERY IN PHYSICAL EDUCATION

Think about your body position as you perform certain skills in class, e.g., kicking a soccer ball, serving a volleyball, doing a cartwheel. What does the position look and feel like? Imagine the body position as clearly as possible. Replay the action forwards and backwards. Observe the movement from the side, front, and rear. Try to imagine the movement again from these differ-ent angles. Share your ideas with the class.

Lie down and observe a partner performing a specific action—walking, skipping, crawling. Imagine what you would look like doing this, imagine what it feels and sounds like. Share your ideas with the class.

IMAGERY LEARNING WORKSHOP

IMAGERY AND SKILL BUILDING

BENEFITS OF IMAGERY

- Ideas come alive
- Control situations
- Plan to act
- Control actions
- Stay calm

Special points of interest:

♦ Imagery is a way to put ourselves in situations that have not happened YET and to make the outcomes successful

♦ Imagery is a pathway, not a solution or destination

♦ Imagery gives the learner a chance to experiment with ideas

♦ Imagination is more important than information

Introduction

This activity focuses on sensing the other features of the environment around the activity. Focus specifically on your response to the environment. In other words, if it is cold outside, sense how you would respond to the cold, e.g., feel the cold air in your lungs, hear the crunch of the snow under your feet.

Before you begin

Lie on your back and use spaghetti activity to get relaxed. When you are quiet and calm, put your hand on your tummy. Feel your breathing. Try to make it a little slower and deeper. Feel your jelly belly rise and fall. Pretend your hand is an air mattress floating on the water.

Activity

Imagine you are jogging through a wooded

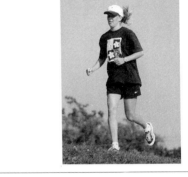

Focus on your response to the environment.

park in the fall. As you begin jogging, you notice the recent rain has made the ground a little wet. What effect does the rain have on the ground? Several branches have fallen and as you approach them you have to react. What will you do to avoid the fallen branches? Leaves are falling around you. As they gently float to the ground what thoughts come to mind? The autumn air is clean, clear, and earthy. How does it feel to breathe and smell the air? How do these sights, sounds, and smells affect the way you are jogging?

USING IMAGERY IN PHYSICAL EDUCATION

When you imagine an activity such as the underhand pass in volleyball or dribbling a basketball, imagine all the other activities happening around you. This helps to make the image 'real.' Imagine your responses to the people around you, your position relative to the net. Imagine the feel of the ball, its texture, weight, and shape as you perform the movements. See and feel in your mind your body in motion. Share your ideas with a partner.

IMAGERY LEARNING WORKSHOP

IMAGERY AND SKILL BUILDING

BENEFITS OF IMAGERY

- Cope with stress
- Change attitude
- Be ready
- Overcome fears
- Accept challenge

Special points of interest:

- Imagery is a way to keep sharp during layoffs. When we aren't practicing or during the off season, it is a good idea to keep in touch with the game through mental imagery activities.

Everyday imagery

- When you have to do things you don't like to do imagine your frustrations, fears, and worries are boulders blocking your way to success. Image them as tiny pebbles and see if you can find ways to overcome them.

Introduction

This activity focuses on making objects change size and shape.

Before you begin

Imagine being invited to have a rest on a bed made of marshmallows. Lay back and feel yourself sink into the marshmallows. Feel the softness wrap around you.

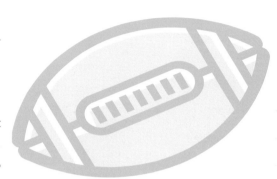

Use imagery to block out distractions and focus on the game.

Activity

Think of an object such as your bed. Imagine that it is getting bigger and bigger. It is so big a giant would look small in it. Imagine inviting your friends over to bounce on this huge bed. Now start to shrink the bed, making it smaller and smaller until it is just big enough for a small mouse.

Try this activity on different objects in the room and on people.

USING IMAGERY IN PHYSICAL EDUCATION

Imagine something that interferes with your performance, e.g. crowd noise, steep hills, an aggressive opponent. Imagine you are able to shrink the interference and enlarge your courage, your determination, and your muscle strength.

Some aboriginal cultures 'tree' their troubles. Just before an event the players place their hands on a tree. They imagine they are putting their worries, rivalries, and stresses into the tree. After the game they can retrieve their troubles (if they want to). This activity is sometimes done after games too so participants will not take their troubles, disappointments, or anger home with them.

Try making the basketball you are working with smaller, lighter, and a soft colour. This might help you feel more comfortable with a regulation size ball.

IMAGERY LEARNING WORKSHOP

IMAGERY AND SKILL BUILDING

BENEFITS OF IMAGERY

- Solve problems
- Concentrate better
- Block distractions
- Relax

Special points of interest:

♦ Use imagery to solve problems
♦ Imagery is a way of authoring your own biography
♦ Imagery can help us change our beliefs and attitudes about ourselves. Sometimes we imagine ourselves poorly. Concentrate on creating images of yourself in a positive light.

Introduction

This activity focuses on creating successful images.

Before you begin

Imagery is the power to reach out to other realities. Can you see yourself as a jet pilot, or an actor on the stage, a person who cares for other people? Take a moment and think about one of these activities.

Activity

*Envision yourself performing one of the skills you are working on in class. See/feel/hear the skill being performed **well.** Try to capture all the good feelings and celebration of a well-executed performance. Before you begin, remind yourself about what the skill should be like when it is done well. What are the key features of a perfect serve, throw, or swing at bat?*

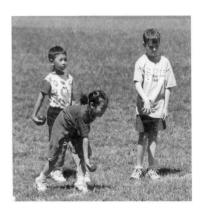

Imagine what it feels and looks like.

USING IMAGERY IN PHYSICAL EDUCATION

When students are practicing a skill, take time before each performance to image the skill and to image a successful performance and outcome. Make the mechanics or form of the skill look and feel good. Enjoy the emotional feelings of success in your imagination too. After each trial, review the action and think again about what makes a high quality performance. It takes mental and physical practice to perform well.

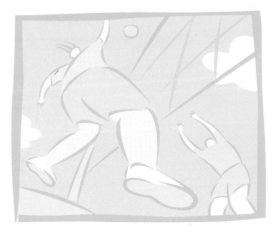

A135

IMAGERY LEARNING WORKSHOP

IMAGERY AND CREATIVITY

BENEFITS OF IMAGERY

BENEFITS OF IMAGERY

- Create new ideas
- Blend ideas
- Test ideas out
- Be innovative

Special points of interest:

- Practice often
- Challenge yourself
- Find new ways to improve learning using imagery
- Be alert to the ways that work best for you

Introduction

To make creative discoveries in imagery it must be possible to recognize meaningful shapes and patterns that emerge from examining images.

Activity

Look at the two Roman numerals.

XX

Now cover them up.
- *How many triangles are there?*
- *Can you see a diamond shape?*
- *Can you find a parallelogram?*
- *Uncover the diagram, how well did you do?*

Repeat the challenge using the number

4

Repeat the challenge above using the Star of David.

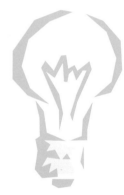

We see great ideas in our heads before we see them in reality.

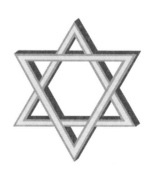

IMAGERY FOR LIFE

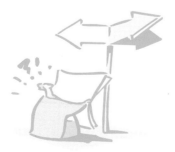

Imagery should become a routine part of the way you think, plan, decide, anticipate, and reflect on activities and events in your life. Seeing in your head is a way to prepare, preplan, and prearrange outcomes.

IMAGERY LEARNING WORKSHOP

IMAGERY AND CREATIVE SKILLS

BENEFITS OF IMAGERY

• Manipulate ideas

• Create new ideas

• Make revisions

Special points of interest:

♦ Try these activities with your family and friends

♦ Make up new challenges

♦ Be inventive/creative

Introduction

This workshop focuses on mentally manipulating familiar symbols.

Activity

Choose two familiar symbols. Close your eyes and combine the two symbols to create a familiar object.

The symbols to choose from are:

☐ , C, J, L, O, 8, X, V, P, D, I, T

Here are some combinations to try:

　　8 and V

　　J and D

　　☐ and P

　　X and C

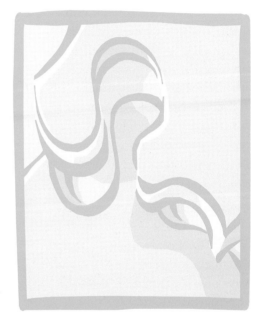

Use imagery to manipulate ideas, to create new ways of doing things.

USING IMAGERY IN PHYSICAL EDUCATION

Movements used in one situation can be transferred to learning other skills. How does the overhand throw relate to the overhand serve in tennis? How does the underhand throw relate to bowling and curling? Look for familiar patterns and relationships between everyday movements and physical activity.

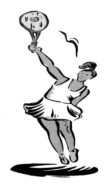

Self-talk

What is self-talk?

Self-talk is like having a coach or teacher in your head cueing your performance. Self-talk can be part of task preparation, execution, follow-up analysis, or the feedback you give yourself to improve. Self-talk is sometimes called private speech, verbal rehearsal, self-instruction or inner voice. Self-talk lets you be your own teacher, guide your own decisions, and remind you about what you are supposed to do to perform well.

Sometimes people use self-talk to help them park their car, look for books in the library, follow a recipe, solve puzzles, overcome fears, and accept new challenges. It is also a powerful learning tool for skill development.

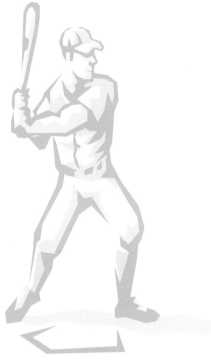

Self-talk is a learning tool.

Benefits of using self-talk:

- Focuses attention on the key elements of performance

- Limits the number of cues that need attention

- Blocks out distractions
- Personalizes learning

- Enables planning, monitoring, and evaluation

- Promotes deliberate action

Gina's story

Gina was worried about going up to bat in front of her classmates. She was afraid they would laugh at her if she struck out. She didn't know how to stand, hold the bat, or swing at the ball. She felt awkward and clumsy. Fortunately, Gina's teacher anticipated these difficulties. He taught Gina to pay attention to two key movements:

1. Stand sideways, hold the bat with your hand nearest the pitcher, pretend to throw a can of pop over your rear shoulder, then bring the other hand up along side the first hand.

2. As the ball approaches pretend to throw your hands at the ball. To help focus on the ball, look at the seams and follow the ball all the way to the bat.

Gina used self-talk to remember what to do, to block out interference, and to feel confident. This is what she said to herself before she went up to bat:

"OK, you know what to do. Sideways, pop over the shoulder, look at the seams, throw hands at the ball."

As the first pitch was delivered you could hear Gina say: "Throw your hands." "Wow, I did it!"

Self-talk

Learning Workshop

Benefits of Self-talk

- Build confidence
- Control anxiety
- Promote precision
- Block distractions

Introduction

What is self-talk good for?

Self-talk Learning Workshop

Show the class a clip from the movie Home Alone. The clip shows the youngster in front of the mirror reminding himself about all the chores he must complete that day. In his adult-like demeanor he combs his hair and finally applies spray deodorant, which generates his trademark scream. Why did the boy in the movie use self-talk in this scene?

Homework

List the benefits of self-talk.
Keep track of times throughout the day when you talk to yourself. Be prepared to share your list in class.

Everyday Self-talk

Self-talk is sometimes a way to think from a different point of view. I can talk pretending to be an announcer on TV or talk like a police officer. Who do you talk like at times?

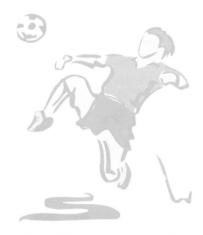

Use self-talk to improve your skills.

Using Self-talk In Physical Education

Self-talk can be used effectively to channel attention towards specific parts of a skill. For the breast stroke: "Remember to glide after the kick" and "Count one - two before starting the arms again." Think of a way to use self-talk in class. Share your ideas.

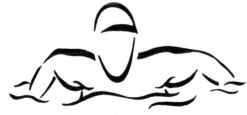

Your inner voice is important.

Self-talk

Learning Workshop

Special points of interest:

- Listen to the way others use self-talk

- Practice using self-talk to guide your actions

- Use self-talk to plan better performances

Introduction
Why do people talk to themselves?

Self-talk Learning Workshop
Keep track of the way other people self-talk. Who could you listen in on?
- teachers
- other students
- parents
- people in stores

Make a list of what people talk to themselves about. Why do they self-talk?

Discuss the conversations and times when people talk to themselves, (e.g., when they are nervous, when the task requires special attention).

Everyday Self-talk
Lots of people talk to themselves when they are in the grocery store picking out food for themselves or others, when they are in the library looking for a book, and when they are following a recipe. List other times when people self-talk.

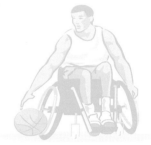

Prepare for action with self-talk.

Using Self-talk In Physical Education

Use self-talk to remember the key parts of a particular skill (e.g., when you catch a ball say, "hands the shape of a basket"). Try it with other skills.

Self-talk Information
Self-talk is a way of connecting new information with what we already know (e.g., "Swing your arm like an elephant's trunk").

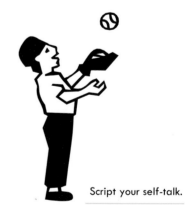

Script your self-talk.

A140

Self-talk

Learning Workshop

Introduction

Self-talk can be used to get 'psyched up' or to calm down.

Self-talk Learning Workshop

Make a list of words or phrases you could say to yourself to boost your confidence and intensity during practice. Pick out one or two of these phrases and see if they increase your ability to play with energy and intensity.

Make a list of words and phrases you could repeat to calm yourself down in tense situations. Share these lists with classmates.

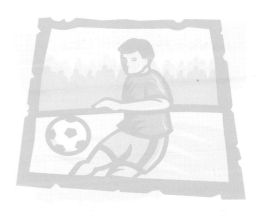

To sharpen focus say, "Look at the spots."

Everyday Self-talk

Some people talk to themselves to hear their ideas out loud.

Using Self-talk In Physical Education

Self-talk can be used to motivate performance. Using words like "Blam!" "Explode" or "Power" can be used to generate energy. Alternatively, self-talk can be used to calm and quiet the mind and body. Words like "soft" and "river flowing" or "melting ice cream" can help keep movements rhythmical and smooth.

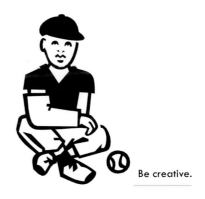

Be creative.

A141

Self-talk

Learning Workshop

Special points of interest:

- Ask friends how they use self-talk

- Listen to what athletes say that suggests they use self-talk too (e.g., "I keep telling myself to focus on the backswing")

Introduction

Self-talkers have a teacher with them at all times. Self-talk should be used to focus on good technique and quality movement patterns.

Self-talk Learning Workshop

Self-talk should focus on aspects of form (e.g., how to hold the equipment, how to position yourself or how to move properly). Self-talk should be about the things you can control — how *you* think, how *you* move, how *you* need to prepare.

Everyday Self-talk

Self-talk is thinking out loud. Self-talk can be a reassuring voice.

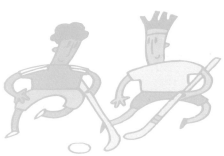

Self-talk is a good way to prepare for an activity.

Using Self-talk In Other Ways

Use self-talk to remind yourself to do the chores around the house. "What would mum and dad want me to do for them? Right, tidy my room and take out the kitty litter, Yuk!"

Using Self-talk In Physical Education

Use self-talk to take better control over your practice time. Work on one or two parts of a skill. Talk yourself through the movements. Practice for quality.

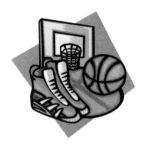

Self-talk

Learning Workshop

Introduction

Some researchers refer to self-talk as inner speech. Always use positive self-talk.

Self-talk Learning Workshop

Positive self-talk is better than negative self-talk. Researchers have found that successful players tend to use more positive self-talk while losers use negative self-talk more often. Try talking to yourself in a positive way. Make a list of positive comments that encourage, boost, and activate learning.

Everyday Self-talk

Untrained self-talkers use negative self-talk often. Planned self-talk should be positive and constructive.

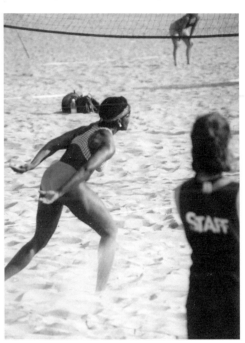

Use self-talk to plan your strategy.

Using Self-talk In Physical Education

Self-talk can be used to maintain effort, persevere, or bounce back from failure.

Be realistic. Talk yourself into doing what is possible: "I know I can dribble with my right hand, let's see if I can talk myself into dribbling with my left hand" or "What am I supposed to remember to do?" or "Don't slap the ball, keep your head up, use the pads of your fingertips—Good work."

Use self-talk to look on the bright side of life!

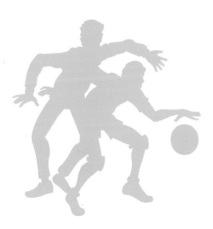

Self-talk

Learning Workshop

Benefits of self-talk

- Boost confidence
- Build skills
- Avoid distractions
- Use as a learning tool

Introduction

Self-talk is like turning up the volume on your inner thoughts and the conversations you have in your head.

Self-talk Learning Workshop

Self-talk can be used to plan or script desired movements. Sometimes self-talk sounds like a pep talk:
"When she serves remember to look at the seams of the ball."
"In this upcoming game concentrate on getting to the ball early. Keep your feet moving."

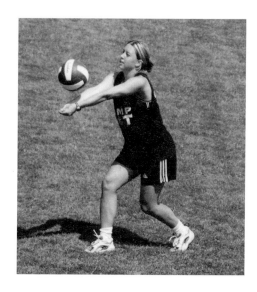

Everyday Self-talk

Is talking in your sleep self-talk? No. Self-talk for improvement should be consciously controlled by the person. Good self-talkers plan to say the 'right' things – words that help them improve.

Self-talk Information

Practice self-talk every day. Practice planning, praising, performing different and difficult tasks using self-talk as a guide, a way to focus, a cheerleader.

Using Self-talk In Physical Education

Use self-talk to boost your level of confidence. Be your own cheerleader. Praise your efforts and achievements. "That was an excellent move. I knew I could do it!" Prepare a script for a skill you are trying to improve. Write a detailed script.

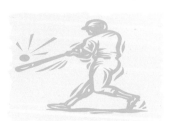

"Throw your hands at the ball."

Self-talk

Learning Workshop

Introduction

Use self-talk with picture words to bring the images alive.

Self-talk Learning Workshop

Picture words can be an important part of self-talk. Picture words are friendlier ways of describing the body action. Using picture words to self-talk may enable learners to remember more information for longer periods of time.

Everyday Self-talk

Use self-talk to organize a piece of writing or to work out a math problem.

Self-talk Information

Develop self-talk scripts that are meaningful for you. Let the teacher help, but YOU decide what words work best!

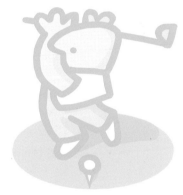

Use self-talk to be in control.

Using Self-talk In Physical Education

Use Self-talk to Build Sports Skills

Use self-talk to guide your performances on the playing field. Identify key parts of the skill, select picture words that describe the body action, and work on mastering the performance. Be your own teacher reminding and reinforcing the skill.

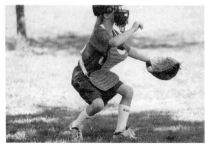

Use positive self-talk.

Self-talk

Learning Workshop

Special points of interest:

- Be your own teacher

- Coach yourself to success

- Praise yourself when you use self-talk well

Introduction
Coordinate self-talk with the body actions.

Self-talk Learning Workshop
Make sure self-talk and the body actions happen at the same time. In other words, say the self-talk words as you are doing or immediately before you do the skill.

Everyday Self-talk
Interview a person in the community to find out if they use self-talk and when.

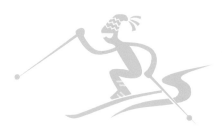

Describe a perfect turn – now do it!

Self-talk Information
When you are using self-talk think of yourself as the teacher and the student. As you self-instruct you will learn important things about learning and teaching.

Using Self-talk In Physical Education

Try this self-talk script for batting. "Stand sideways, throw a can of pop over your shoulder, throw your hands at the ball, twist out from underneath your shoulders as you swing." Now give it a try! Do it as you say it.

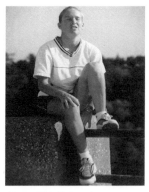

Use self-talk to rehearse and review.

Self-talk

Learning Workshop

Special points of interest:

- Identify what parts you want to improve

- Spend time each day using self-talk to improve

- Listen to 'yourself-talk'

- Make self-talk positive and progressive

Introduction

Speak directly to the body parts you are focusing on.

Self-talk Learning Workshop

Talking to body parts works, too. Talk to your feet, for example - tell them what they are supposed to do.

Praise them when they work well, too. For example, "Feet look straight ahead, good!" "Now jump to the ball and use 'big foot' (wide part of the inside of your foot) to kick the ball."

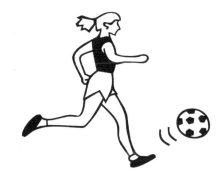

Self-talk Information

Plan what you are going to say. Develop a script for what you want to say to yourself to perform well.

Using Self-talk In Physical Education

For whatever skill you are working on, identify a body part and movement that needs improvement. Use self-talk to improve a specific performance. Speak directly to the body parts that are performing the action. For example, "Throw your hands at the ball when you are up to bat!" "Hands get ready!" "Good hands!"

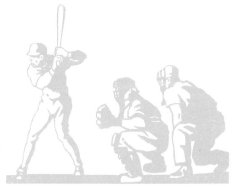

Use self-talk to block out distractions.

Self-talk

Learning Workshop

Special points of interest:

- Self-talk scripts must be carefully planned

- Choose the words that are meaningful, positive, and clear

- Emphasize quality outcomes, e.g., for batting say: " throw your hands at the ball," NOT "I've got to hit a home run"

Introduction
Self-talk can be used to boost your confidence and inspire peak performances.

Self-talk Learning Workshop
Use self-talk to reassure yourself. For example: "OK, this is a shot you can make. What are you supposed to do to shoot the puck well? Can you see the shot in your head? Can you feel it in your arms? Good, you have a lot of knowledge about this skill. Take a deep breath and show them your skills."

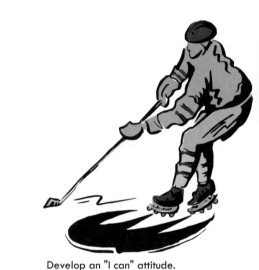

Develop an "I can" attitude.

Using Self-talk In Physical Education

Practice using self-talk to prepare for and execute quality performances. Set aside time to polish skills and the self-talk that goes with them to make a complete mental and physical package.
Don't talk too much. Keep the conversation to a few words. Pick words or phrases that are meaningful: "Racquet back fast!" "Step off back foot!"
Praise your achievements: "Right on!"

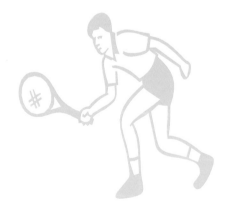

Self-talk

Learning Workshop

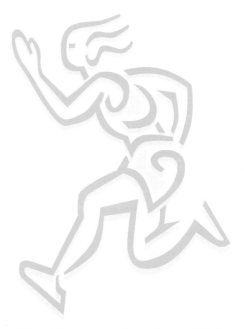

Special points of interest:

- Make self-talk conversational during the preparation phase and then convert the script into short cues during performance.

- Afterwards, use self-talk to analyze the performance.

Introduction

Make self-talk conversational. Self-talk is your inside teacher, coach, and cheerleader.

Self-talk Learning Workshop

Use self-talk to ask questions.
Q. #1 What am I supposed to do to sprint well?
Q. #2 What did the instructor say?
"Oh, right, run tall, arms by your side, knees high, stay on your toes. OK, try that on the next run."
Q. #3 How good did that feel?

Homework

Interview athletes to find out what questions they ask themselves and when they use self-talk. Share your results in class.

What skills are you going to improve? Make self-talk part of the plan.

Using Self-talk In Physical Education

Select a skill you need to improve. Decide what the key components of performance are and then develop a self-talk script. Put your plans into action. Keep track of your progress and report on your successes. Develop three key questions you need to ask yourself.

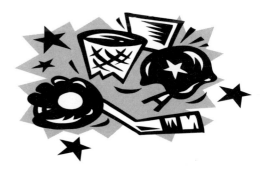

Self-talk

Learning Workshop

Self-talk

Learning Workshop

Special points of interest:

- Self-talk should be positive and used before AND after performance.

- Keep the praise simple and focused on the quality of your movements, e.g., "Yes! I really hit that ball squarely in the centre of the racquet."

Introduction

Include praise and pats on the back for yourself. Self-talk should build skills and confidence.

Self-talk Learning Workshop

Don't forget to praise yourself using self-talk. "I did that well." "Good ball control."

Everyday Self-talk

Take time everyday to look at your accomplishments and praise your successes no matter how small. "I worked hard on that skill. I really can learn difficult skills when I put my mind to it."

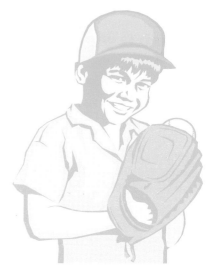

Keeping the target in mind is important, but focusing on what has to be done to hit the target is critical.

Using Self-talk In Physical Education

Include praise in your plans for skill building. Ask yourself: "How would the teacher or coach give you positive feedback?" "Right on!" "Excellent!"

Self-talk Information

High achievers rely on their own feedback to help them make clear and precise decisions.

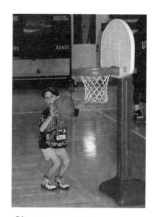

Plan your route to success.

Self-talk

Learning Workshop

Introduction

Say what you need to say to be successful. Keep it simple and straightforward.

Self-talk Learning Workshop

Don't talk too much. Use one- or two-word phrases when you self-talk, unless there is a lot of time. To increase stride length for skating say: "Stretch the stride."
Then praise:
"Good stuff!"
Reflect on the performance:
"I could really feel my speed increase!"

Special points of interest:

- Continue to polish the use of self-talk and the scripts you use to improve your skills.

- Change your training program to reflect different phases of your development.

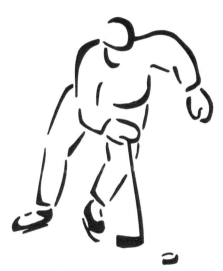

Choose self-talk that is easy to remember and use it when you need It.

Using Self-talk In Physical Education

Select two or three key words you can use to self-talk and improve a particular skill. For throwing a football:

Grip: "spiderweb fingers"
Stance: "stand sideways"
Ready to throw: "statue arm"

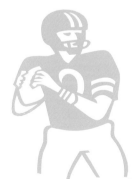

Keep the script short and simple.

Goal-setting

Learning workshop

Introduction

When you got out of bed in the morning, how did you decide what to wear to school?

How are your actions connected to your goals? What do you expect to do today? Making plans is part of goal-setting.

The first steps in goal-setting involve finding out if the main goal can be developed in parts. What are the important parts of walking, writing a story, cleaning your room?

Throughout the day, keep track of instances where you have to accomplish something and, in order to do it well, you have to perform a series of smaller steps.

Goal-setting is natural. We set mini-goals all the time to accomplish various tasks. Make a list of goals - short-term goals. Think of the smaller steps that are part of progress toward those goals.

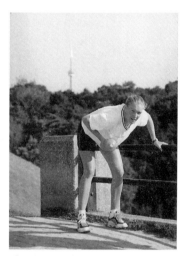

Goals must be realistic and specific to your needs.

Benefits of goal-setting:

- To focus
- To plan for improvement
- To motivate

USING GOAL-SETTING IN PHYSICAL EDUCATION

Select a skill you would like to improve. Identify important parts of the skill you can focus on individually.

Use the goal-setting sheet to plan your progress.

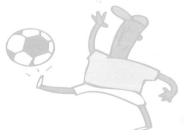

Plan to succeed.

GOAL-SETTING

LEARNING WORKSHOP

Introduction

Use the SMART approach to goal-setting:

S = specific

M = measurable

A = attainable

R = realistic

T = time limited

This workshop focuses on setting specific goals.

Learning Workshop

Set specific goals. For example, I want to improve my running speed. To improve speed I must improve my strength and running skills. Specifically, I will focus on:

• Running tall

• Knees waist height

• Arms beside the body

• Look down the track 20 m

To build strength in my upper legs I will practice the wall sit for 2 minutes each day.

I will practice running for speed 3 times a week. Keep track of progress.

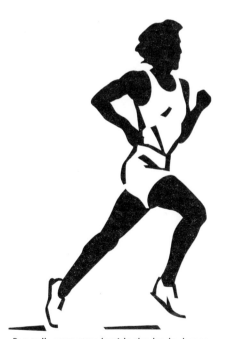

Run tall, arms stay beside the body, knees waist height.

Special points of interest:

• Choose specific goals

• Concentrate on quality

• Practice with goals in mind

• Review goals often

GOAL-SETTING

LEARNING WORKSHOP

Introduction

Make goals that are measurable.

Learning workshop

Goals that are measurable are easier to track, review and keep in focus.

For example:

- I want to improve my shooting by 10%.

- I will make sure that I look at the eyelits on the rim 8 out of 10 times.

- I will self-talk at least once during my time on the floor.

- I will add two more pushups to my workout every week.

- I will spend 15 minutes each day practicing my shot from around the key.

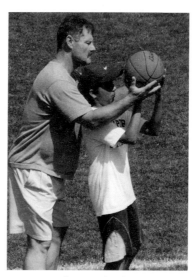

Eyes on the rim.

Special points of interest:

- Identify goals that are important to improvement

- How can you measure your improvement?

- Practice towards specific improvements

USING GOAL-SETTING IN PHYSICAL EDUCATION

Select a skill and identify two measurable goals that would improve performance. Try to reach these goals.

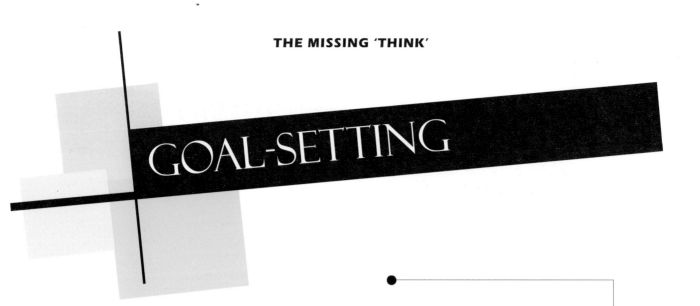

GOAL-SETTING

LEARNING WORKSHOP

Introduction

Select goals that are attainable.

Learning workshop

Both short-and long-term goals that are attainable result in the best improvements. Long-term goals might be: I want to swim two lengths of the pool. Short-term goals focus on improving for example, arm action, kicking, and breathing.

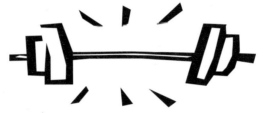

Improve day by day towards long-term goals.

Avoid goals that are focused only on outcomes: I want to beat my opponent. Select goals that are focused on performance: I want to improve my forehand.

Special points of interest:

- Choose goals that are focused on improvements in performance

- Choose goals that are specific

USING GOAL-SETTING IN PHYSICAL EDUCATION

Select a skill you want to improve - identify long- and short-term goals. For example:

Long-term goal

develop a better serve

Short-term goals

- toss the ball as if you were lifting an ice-cream cone

- scratch your back as you prepare to swing

- make contact in the centre of the racquet

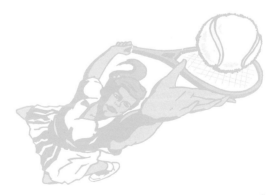

Goals focus effort.

GOAL-SETTING

LEARNING WORKSHOP

Introduction

Select goals that are realistic.

Learning Workshop

Goals that are realistic are more likely to be achieved.

Goals like "I want to play in the NHL" or "I want to score more goals than any other player on the team" may not be realistic. These goals lack details about how to achieve them.

It is better to focus on goals that are realistic in terms of your age and stage of development. If you are just learning a skill, focus on quality. If you are polishing a skill, focus on details that will result in high levels of performance.

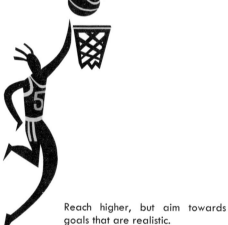

Reach higher, but aim towards goals that are realistic.

Special points of interest:

- Select goals that YOU can achieve

- Choose goals suited to your age and stage of development

- Review goals often

- Detail what you want to improve

USING GOAL-SETTING IN PHYSICAL EDUCATION

Write down goals you have for improving a skill you are working on in class. Be sure the goals are realistic. Share them with a friend and discuss how you can design your practices accordingly.

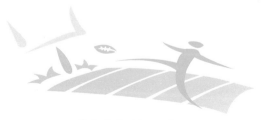

Set attainable goals.

GOAL-SETTING

LEARNING WORKSHOP

Introduction

Select goals that are time limited.

Learning workshop

Goals that are immediate, that is, achievable within the next few days, are more likely to be attained than goals that are remote. Although it is important to have a few long range goals, goals that are close in terms of time will fuel your enthusiasm for improvement and keep you focused.

Time limited goals might include:

I want to improve my high jump skills. Over the next week, I will concentrate on my approach. To-

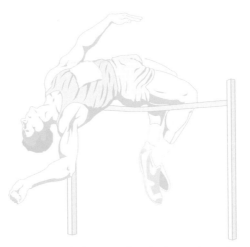

Select goals that are close in time to keep focused.

day, I will carefully calculate the exact number of steps and where I should start from to ensure a consistent run-up to the bar.

Special points of interest:

• Select goals that can be achieved soon

• Practice with specific performance details in mind

• Be realistic – learning is a complex process

USING GOAL-SETTING IN PHYSICAL EDUCATION

Identify a performance goal you can achieve in this class. For example, in class today, I want to work on making sure I get behind the ball when I underhand pass the volleyball. I want to be able to do that at least 3 out of 5 tries.

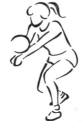

Record Progress.

GOAL-SETTING

LEARNING WORKSHOP

This workshop focuses on developing goals for a walking program. This example shows how goal setting can improve performance and achievement.

Mary and David decided they wanted to start a walking program to improve their health. The first step was to develop good walking technique. During their first walk they focused on walking tall, a comfortable stride, proper heel toe foot contact and a smooth arm swing. Both made sure they wore comfortable (low heeled) shoes. Mary used self-talk to remind herself to align her body like building blocks. David used imagery to remember to relax (float) as he walked. After all, this was supposed to be good for his mental and physical health.

Every other evening they set out for a 2 km walk. After 2 weeks they increased the distance to 3 km. David and Mary want to set some goals that would give them an incentive and reward for their dedication. Mary wants to be able to walk around Wolfe Island. David wants to be able to participate in a 10 km walk for cancer. They put together a plan that would give them variety in their route and progressive increases in distance and challenge over different terrain. This is their schedule for the next month.

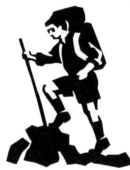

"The length of my walk is the length of my thought."
Thoreau

Special points of interest:

- Set realistic goals

- Set specific goals

- Set goals in relation to your improvement

- Keep track of your progress

USING GOAL-SETTING IN PHYSICAL EDUCATION

Week 1: walk around park (4 km) (M, W,F,S)

Week 2: walk to the museum and back along the river path (5 km) (M,T,T,S,S)

Week 3: walk to the school track (6 km) (M,T,W,F,S)

Week 4: walk to the old church (6.5 km) in less than 50 minutes. (M,T,W,F,S)

Enjoy the scenery too!

Bibliography

Afremow, J., Overby, L., & Vadocz, E. (1996). *Using mental imagery to enhance the sport and dance skills of children.* East Lansing, MI: Michigan State University.

Anderson, A. (1997). Learning strategies in physical education: Self-talk, imagery, and goal-setting. *Journal of Physical Education, Recreation, and Dance*, 68 (1), 30-35.

Anderson, A. (1992). Using self-talk as a strategy for learning the overhand throw. Unpublished doctoral dissertation, Michigan State University.

Anderson, A. & Goode, R. (1997). Assessment informs instruction. *Journal of Physical Education, Recreation, and Dance*, 68 (3), 42-49.

Armstrong, C. A., Sallis, J. F., Hovell, M. F., & Hofstetter, C. R. (1993). Stages of change, self-efficacy, and the adoption of vigorous exercise: A prospective analysis. *Journal of Sport & Exercise Psychology*, 15, 390-402.

Arsanow, J. R. & Meichenbaum, D. (1979). Verbal rehearsal and serial recall: The meditational training of kindergarten children. *Child Development*, 50, 1173-1177.

Beimiller, A. & Meichenbaum, D. (1992). The nature and nurture of the self-directed learner. *Educational Leadership*, October, 75-80.

Bershad, C. & DiMella, N. (1984). How teens can make their self-talk positive. *PTA Today*, 9, 15-16.

Brown, A. L. & Palinscar, A. (1989). Guided cooperative learning and individual knowledge acquisition. In L. B. Resnick (Ed.), *Knowing, learning, and instruction: Essays in honor of Robert Glaser* (pp. 393-452). Hillsdale, NJ: Erlbaum.

Bunker, L. K., Williams, J. M., & Zinsser, N. (1993). Cognitive techniques for improving performance and building confidence. In J. M. Williams (Ed.), *Applied sport psychology: Personal growth to peak performance* (pp. 198-214). Mountain View, CA: Mayfield.

Burton, D. (1992). The Jekyll/Hyde nature of goals: Reconceptualizing goal setting in sport. In T. Horn (Ed.), *Advances in Sport Psychology* (pp. 267-297). Champaign, IL: Human Kinetics.

Chi, M. T. H. & Bassok, M. (1989). Learning from examples via self-explanations. In L. B. Resnick (Ed.), *Knowing, learning, and instruction: Essays in honor of Robert Glaser* (pp. 251-282). Hillsdale, NJ: Erlbaum.

Chi, M., De Leeuw, N., Chiu, M-H., & LaVancher, C. (1994). Eliciting self-explanations improves understanding. *Cognitive Science*, 18, 439-477.

Csikszentmihalyi, M. (1990). *Flow: The psychology of optimal performance.* New York: Harper & Row.

Docherty, D. (1975). *Education through dance experience.* Bellingham, WA: Educational Designs and Consultants.

Englert, C. S., Raphael, T., Anderson, L., Anthony, H., & Stevens, D. (1991). Making strategies and self-talk visible: Writing instruction in regular and special education classrooms. *American Educational Research Journal*, 28, 337-372.

Feltz, D. L. (1982). The effects of age and number of demonstrations on modeling of form and performance. *Research Quarterly for Exercise and Sport*, 53, 291-296.

Fuson, K. C. (1979). The development of self-regulating aspects of speech: A review. In G. Zivin (Ed.), *The development of self-regulation through private speech* (pp. 135-217). New York: Wiley.

Gould, D. & Weiss, M. (1981). The effects of model similarity and model talk on self-efficacy and muscular endurance. *Journal of Sport Psychology*, 3, 17-29.

Jones, B. F., Palinscar, A., Ogle, D., & Carr, E. (1987). *Strategic teaching and learning: Cognitive instruction in the content areas.* Alexandria, VA: Association for Supervision and Curriculum Development.

Hawkins, D. (1974). I, thou, it. In *The informed vision: Essays on learning and human nature* (pp. 48-62). New York: Agallion Press.

Landin, D. (1994). The role of verbal cues in skill learning. *Quest*, 46, 299-313.

Lang, P. J., Kozak, M., Miller, G. A., Lavin, B., & McLean, A. (1980). Emotional imagery: Conceptual structure and pattern of somato-visceral response. *Psychophysiology*, 17, 179-192.

Locke, E. A., Shaw, K. N., Saari, L. M., & Latham, G. P. (1981). Goal setting and task performance: 1969-1980. *Psychological Bulletin*, 90, 125-152.

Locke, E. A. & Latham, G. P. (1985). The application of goal setting to sports. *Journal of Sports Psychology*, 7, 205-222.

Marcus, B. H., Selby, V. C., Niaura, R. S., & Rossi, J. S. (1992). Self-efficacy and the stage of exercise behaviour change. *Research Quarterly for Exercise and Sport*, 63, 60-66.

McCullagh, P., Stiehl, J., & Weiss, M. (1990). Developmental modeling effects on the quantitative and qualitative aspects of motor performance. *Research Quarterly for Exercise and Sport*, 61, 344-350.

Meichenbaum, D. & Beimiller, A. (1990). In search of student expertise in the classroom: A metacognitive analysis. Paper presented at the conference on cognitive research for instructional innovation, University of Maryland, College Park, Maryland, May 10.

Meichenbaum, D. (1977). *Cognitive-behavior modification: An integrative approach*. New York: Plenum.

Michigan's Exemplary Physical Education Curriculum. (1995). *Program and Instructional Objectives for Physical Education*. Spring Arbor, MI: Michigan Fitness Foundation. (Available from Michigan Fitness Foundation, P.O. Box 27187, Lansing, MI, 48909).

Murphy, S. & Jowdy, D. (1992). Imagery and mental practice. In T. Horn (Ed.), *Advances in Sport Psychology*. Human Kinetics.

Orlick, T. & Partington, J. (1988). Mental links to excellence. *The Sport Psychologist*, 2, 105-130.

Orlick, T. (1986). *Psyching for sport: Mental training for athletes*. Champaign, IL: Leisure Press.

Peterson, P. L. & Swing, S. (1983). Problems in classroom implementation of cognitive instruction. In M. Pressley & J. Levin (Eds.), *Cognitive strategy research: Educational applications* (pp. 267-288). New York: Springer-Verlag.

Sage, G. H. (1984). *Motor learning and control: A neuropsychological approach*. Dubuque, IA: Wm. C. Brown.

Scheid, K. (1995). *Helping students become strategic learners*. Cambridge: Brookline Books.

Schonfeld, A. H. (1983). Beyond the purely cognitive: Belief systems, social cognitions, and metacognitions as driving forces in intellectual performance. *Cognitive Science*, 7, 329-363.

Schunk, D. H. (1991). *Learning theories: An educational perspective*. New York: Macmillan.

Schunk, D. (1986). Self-regulation through overt verbalization during cognitive skill learning. *Contemporary Educational Psychology*, 77 (3), 347-369.

Shasby, G. (1986). Improving movement skills through language. *Motor skills: Theory into practice*, Vol. 7 (1-2), 91-96.

Singer, R. (1986, April). Sport performance: A five-step approach. *Journal of Physical Education, Recreation, and Dance*, 13-17.

Smith, (1991). Where is the child in physical education research? *Quest*, 43, 37-54.

Suinn, R.M. (1980). Psychology and sport performance: Principles and applications. In R. Suinn (Ed.), *Psychology in sports: Methods and applications* (pp. 26-36). Minneapolis: Burgess.

Thomas, J. R., Lochbaum, M. R., Landers, D. M., & He, C. (1997). Planning significant and meaningful research in exercise science: Estimating sample size. *Research Quarterly for Exercise and Sport*, 68, 33-43.

Vogel, P. & Seefeldt, V. (1990). *Performance criteria and rating scale: The overhand throw.* East Lansing, MI: Michigan State University. Unpublished document.

Van Raalte, J. L., Brewer, B. W., Rivera, P. M., & Petitpas, A. J. (1994). The relationship between observable self-talk and competitive junior tennis players' match performance. *Journal of Sport and Exercise Psychology*, 16, 400-415.

Vermunt, J. D. (1987). Regulation of learning, approaches to studying, and learning styles of adult students. In P. R. Simons & G. Beukof (Eds.), *Regulation of learning* (pp. 15-32). The Hague: S.V.O.

Vygotsky, L.S. (1962). *Thought and language.* Cambridge, MA: M.I.T. Press. (Original work published 1934).

Weaver, R. L. & Cotrell, H. (1987). Destructive dialogue: Negative self-talk and effective imaging. Paper presented at the annual meeting on the speech communication association (73rd, Boston, MA, Nov. 5-8).

Weiss, M. R. (1983). Modeling and motor performance: A developmental perspective. *Research Quarterly for Exercise and Sport*, 54, 190-197.

Weiss, M. R. & Klint, K. A. (1987). "Show and tell" in the gymnasium: An investigation of developmental differences in modeling and verbal rehearsal of motor skills. *Research Quarterly for Exercise and Sport*, 58, 234-241.

West, C. K., Farmer, J., & Wolff, P. (1991). *Instructional design: Implications from cognitive science.* Englewood Cliffs, NJ: Prentice-Hall.

Weinstein. C. E. & Mayer, R. (1986). The teaching of learning strategies. In M. C. Wittrock (Ed.), *Handbook of research on teaching* (pp. 315-328). New York: MacMillan.

Williams, J. M. & Leffingwell, T. R. (1996). Cognitive strategies in sport and exercise psychology. In Van Raalte & Brewer (Eds.), *Exploring sport and exercise psychology.* Washington, D. C.: American Psychological Association.

Winne, P. H. (1985). Cognitive processing in the classroom. In T. Husen & T. N. Postlewaite (Eds.), *The international encyclopedia of education* (Vol. 2, pp. 795-808). Oxford, England: Pergamon Press.

About the Author

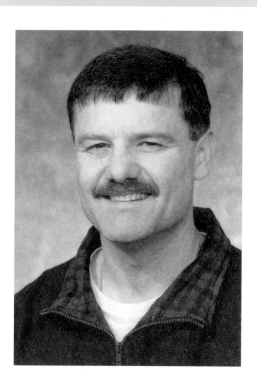

Andy Anderson is an associate professor at the Ontario Institute for Studies in Education at the University of Toronto. As a teacher, physical and health education consultant, and teacher educator at the faculty of education, he has always been a strong supporter of student involvement in the learning process. "Equipped with tools for learning, students are more engaged and, as a result, can lead the way to their understanding." At the graduate level, he has been involved in teacher preparation programs around the world. His most recent work has been in Thailand teaching graduate courses for Michigan State University. His workshops on learning strategy use have been presented at national and international conferences, local school districts, and summer teacher development programs. In 1998, Andy was a recipient of the distinguished teaching award for arts and humanities from the University of Toronto. The Missing 'Think' is the result of over 10 years of academic and practice-based study of learning strategy use in physical education and coaching settings.